Courageous Birth

THE JOYS & CHALLENGES OF FULLY EMBRACING PREGNANCY, HOME BIRTH & BABIES

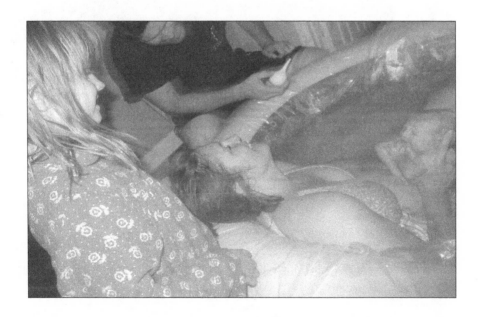

DR. LAURA SIMS D.C.

1ST EDITION

Courageous Birth By Dr. Laura Sims D.C.

Published 2020 by Your Book Angel

Copyright © Dr. Laura Sims D.C.

Printed in the United States

Edited by Keidi Keating

Layout by Rochelle Mensidor

ISBN: 978-1-7341814-7-0

CONTENTS

I'd like to dedicate this to
Grace, Ada, Rae & Finley Rose.
This wouldn't be possible if it weren't for them.

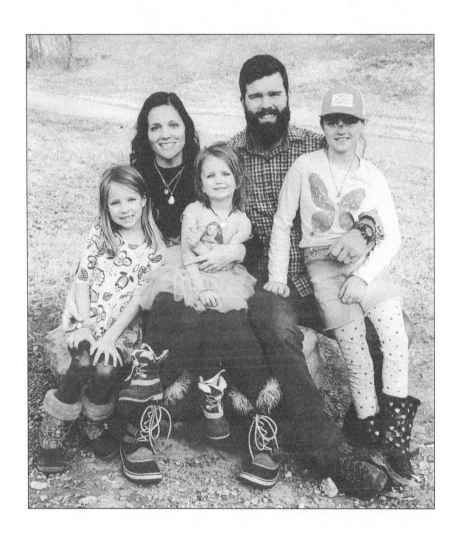

INTRODUCTION

Why am I writing this?

It all began as my Spiritual Psychology 2nd year Master's program "sacred yes" project. When I was pregnant for the first time in 2008, I scoured the library and internet for information on home birth. It was disappointing at best. There have been women having babies at home since the beginning of time. "Why is there not an enormous database on home birth?" I thought to myself. I found *Spiritual Midwifery* and a couple of other interesting books on the topic. Nothing that completely resonated with me. Ina May's *Guide to Childbirth* was the most helpful.

This book is a compilation of everything I was yearning for at that time in my life: a woman's personal experience with pregnancy, home water birth and starting a family. Something non-clinical, authentic and real. I realize the amount of information available now on the topic of home water birth and natural birth is a lot more. My intention with *Courageous Birth* is to leave this legacy for my daughters and their daughters and all of our daughters to know that no matter the challenges that arise, you are not alone.

This book can be used in many ways. You can read it from start to finish. Or you can go directly to the chapter that applies to what you're going through at this time in your life. I don't hold back as it pertains to my experiences. This may be TMI for some, and super helpful for those that are searching for answers and really need those details. With whatever stage of life you are in, my intention is to relay my experience in service to you. I want you to benefit in some way from this real, raw version of pregnancy, birth and tragedy. When it came to writing the final chapters, I wondered if it was too much. Too much for me? Too much for others to read about? I thought about it and I decided that part of the reason I had those experiences was to help others who are also going through them, to comfort others in their greatest time of need, and to be real. No matter what you're going though, just know that there is an opportunity here. An opportunity for growth and learning. An opportunity for healing. Opportunities for living into who God made you to be. Freeing yourself from the misidentifications, misbeliefs, judgements, limitations, resentments and un-forgiveness.

With Gratitude

I write my first book today and I feel like I was made to write this. Really, there's never the "perfect" time for when you're 100% ready to write, conceive a child or dive into your sacred yes. Here's my story...

1

SURPRISES
IN LIFE

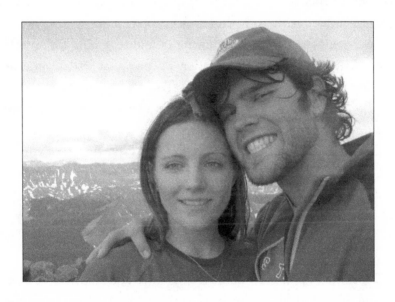

The best things happen unexpectedly...

Young, happy and following our dreams. That was Jacob and
I. Married for 5 years now, both graduated as Doctors of
Chiropractic and driving for the last time from Georgia to

where we would be starting our life in Colorado. It was December 2007 when we pulled into Crested Butte with all of our worldly possessions and 2 dogs. We moved into our new home, a condo above a gas station. It felt amazing! It was in a blizzard, but it didn't matter. We had followed our dreams and had decided to live and open up our office in a town of 1,500. This is where we wanted to end up and were determined to make the business succeed while enjoying our lives!

The decision to live in Crested Butte came recently, during Jacob's final quarter. Prior, we had intended to open in Denver area. So there we were, just going for it.

I instantly fell in love with this beautiful place. Our condo, recently renovated, felt spacious and nice. Especially compared to our living situation in college, where we were in an outdated town home with puke green tiled bathrooms and broken appliances.

We spent the days ahead moving in and searching for an office space. After looking at every option in town, we settled on a new building in the center of town. Our office was required to be on the 2nd floor per town rules regarding the main street. Things were moving fast!

My youngest brother was getting married shortly after we moved and I went to Denver for the wedding. I was a bridesmaid. I thought I'd be the youngest of everyone as far as age when I got married, but he beat me. He was actually 17 when he and his wife eloped. They are still married to this day! The wedding in Denver was the big, fancy church wedding.

I returned to our new home feeling alive and ready for what was coming with starting our business in this majestic place. Jacob and I had a fun and loving reunion on January 8, 2008.

Given our large amount of student loan debt and the fact that all we had to start our business was the $11,000 I'd saved working prior to college as well as an interest-free credit card with a $7,000 dollar limit that didn't have to be paid back for a year, we got to work immediately! We made our office space nice. I noticed I was feeling a bit crazy and chalked it up to all the preparations for this new office and starting it. "Feels like a lot," I thought. With much enthusiasm and excitement, we opened our doors. People actually came in to see us! It was amazing and all so surreal.

I noticed it was more challenging to breathe when I'm out on my walks and runs. I figured it was the altitude. It is 9,000 feet. Then, I almost vomited when opening the fridge and chili smells greeted my hypersensitive nasal passages. A food I normally devour was now making me feel like vomiting even though I hadn't eaten a single bite. "Weird," I thought. I went about my life thinking this would pass, but it just wasn't passing! Jacob hinted that maybe I was pregnant. I emphatically denied that even being a possibility. We were using a condom the days I was fertile, right? Apparently my cycle had become sporadic with the move and the wedding and all the shenanigans. I didn't think it was possible that I was pregnant, but I could not go one more second without knowing.

On February 16, 2008, I went to Clark's Market and grabbed my first pregnancy test ever. I needed to know, NOW! I peed on the stick and let it sit on the counter. It immediately produced a pink plus sign. No denying it. I took another test, thinking the first might have been defective. Same result. Where was Jacob, you might ask? On top of a 12,000 foot mountain overlooking the town. I said to myself, "Why didn't I wait to pee on the stick until he was back?" I had felt that it would be a disappointment if it had been negative. I thought, "I can't get his hopes up, just to be dashed in the event I'm not pregnant." Now, I phoned him and said, "I took a pregnancy test and it's positive. I'm PREGNANT! What are we going to do?" He was overjoyed. I was in shock. And so the adventure began…

Three days later I told him I knew exactly how I wanted to give birth: a home water birth. I just knew it was going to be incredible and I had his full backing. We told all of our family and friends. It was the 1st grandchild on both sides. Everyone was excited and some were concerned about our home birth choice. I already had a list of all the items I needed: blow-up pool, cord ring, fetoscope, suction bulb, etc.

Did I mention we had just started our business? Heh. Yeah. We were newly opened and I was pregnant.

I headed for the library. It's likely the tiniest library in the world. I was able to order in every single home birth book out at the time. Not a whole lot of choices. Things like *Ina May's Guide to Childbirth*, *Sacred Midwifery*, *The Bradley Method*, and a couple water birth books. From everything, I found Ina May Gaskin to be the best resource. She has such a rich history on The Farm and dozens of testimonials of home birth. She was such a wealth of knowledge that was so helpful and uplifting to me.

We had lots of amazing outdoor opportunities with lots of snowboarding in Colorado. So we decided to hike and snowboard down the neighboring mountains—cornices that were enormous as well as lots and lots of powder. That winter, it snowed daily for 2 months solid, and it continued to snow quite frequently through May. The sidewalks were like tunnels, with snow piled higher than a one-story building. Our dogs had to tunnel through feet of snow every time we let them out. It was a winter wonderland. I did all of this activity pregnant and felt fantastic. Yes, I really felt good. Not always the case as you'll read about with future pregnancies.

I was super active with hiking and snowboarding as well as teaching a weekly Pilates class, and needing to pee *all* the time. Surprisingly, the first trimester involves having to urinate frequently, even in the middle of the night, due to all the processes going on within the body, more than any other phase of pregnancy.

At the beginning of April I felt butterfly sensations in my belly. I felt this human moving inside of me for the first time! I was 14 or 15 weeks along.

I was up in the middle of the night at random—no rhyme or reason—thinking about what it was going to be like to give birth and have a child. I was feeling major food aversions and I couldn't take the smell of coffee or bacon or eggs or anything for that matter. I remember thinking about whether I was having a boy or a girl. Most everyone said they thought boy while Jacob had a feeling it was a girl. We harvested wood for a crib that he was building out of beautiful logs.

I had baby names listed: Tristan Ray, Ethny Grace or Ada Grace. We decided we were not going to name the new baby until we had a bit of time together after the birth. We wanted to spend some time with new baby first.

I constructed a birthing plan, basically consisting of how I wanted privacy and a completely supportive environment that was quiet, dark and void of distractions. I like to prepare as much as I can before I do anything. Important to note: Things doesn't always go according to plan. I do, however, believe you can achieve what you set out to do, with the proper team of people around you and a solid belief in your body's abilities.

Nesting became a thing in the 3rd trimester. I wanted to make sure everything was ready for baby. Cleaning became obsessive along with making sure I had everything I'd need for the birth and a new baby. We didn't have a lot of money, but my mom threw a baby shower for us. There were a lot of folks I didn't even know that were her friends. It was nice of everyone to fulfill the registry we'd put together. Being a first-time mom, I had no idea what I really needed. I basically put a lot of things on the list from a multitude of categories.

I feel the need to lay out the only things you really, actually need. The essentials include:

- Diapers
- A changing station situation (for us, this was simply a changing pad we placed on top of an existing dresser)
- Swaddles (I find the Velcro kind to be the simplest as they require no special skills to get on)
- Bibs
- Burp cloths
- Baby bath towel
- Car seat
- Baby carrier (I liked the ergo baby carrier)
- Boppy nursing pillow, which is also handy for them to be propped up on

- Onesie outfits (I need to add a note on this regarding dressing a newborn because this type of attire is key. I attempted to put all sorts of pant/top, dresses and other outfits that were so challenging to get off and on. The baby will have blowouts and spit-ups multiple times a day that require regular outfit changes. Make it easy on yourself and grab some zip-up onesies!)
- Breast pump, bottles and milk bags if you plan on having help in the night or during the day with feedings.
- Bumbo seat with tray for when they start to eat solids
- Optional:
- Bassinet, crib or whatever bed scenario you desire. We actually used neither of these with baby #1 because we co-slept
- Stroller (comes in handy with more than one child)

I was adjusting patients up until the very end of my pregnancy. I got a lot of unsolicited commentary on my pregnancy. "Are you sure you aren't having twins?" and "You're having your baby at home?!" and "What if something goes wrong?" and "I knew someone who had a home birth and the baby died from inhaling meconium," and "You're carrying high so that baby won't be coming for a while," and "It's a boy because you are just glowing," and "It's definitely a girl because of the shape of your belly," and on and on. I put a lot of pressure on myself to appear like everything was fine, even though I was feeling quite large and was not okay with some of the commentary. I just brushed it off. That's what I did at that time in my life and leading up to that pregnancy. My motto was: You don't tell people what you're actually feeling because it's not nice.

All along, I was thinking about how awesome it was going to be and trusting myself and my body. I knew it would go well and that my body was made for this! I continued to be active. Walking, hiking, rafting, fishing, camping and Pilates happened often. I felt really great physically. And very large.

It was September and the "due date" was the 30th. I happened to meet a doula named Annie. It felt like divine timing for her to enter the picture. She was going to be there to assist me during the birth and after. She had been to one birth in her experience as a doula and she was just starting her dream to help mothers while in the throes of labor and after. Annie and I met a couple of times and I was feeling solid with how the birth process was going to be. I also felt extremely empowered by all the birth stories I had read in *Spiritual Midwifery* and the other birth books. At this point, I realized my potential and my strength! The events leading up to this birth were all in service to my learning and readying myself for birth.

The place we live is so enlivening and majestic. I was discovering more and more of this small mountain town. Walking daily at this point and hiking was helping me stay sane. There were so many days I wrote to the baby in my belly. I journaled to the baby. I talked to baby. I loved her even before I knew she was a her.

My September 18, 2008 journal entry talks about having Braxton-Hicks contractions. "Clearly the big day will be soon," I wrote. I wrote about Jacob and his long hair and ponytail, and how much lower in my pelvis baby felt. I was able to breathe a bit easier once that happened!

It was the end of the month, and still no baby. I became ill. I had a fever, a wicked cough and aches all over. I hadn't been sick in 2 years and now I felt like I was going to die when I was right up against the biggest thing I had ever done in my entire life—this marathon called birth. I took 3 days straight to just rest.

I found out my friend, whom I'd been pregnant with and spent time with, had had her baby. Her birth had ended in a C-section. Things were progressing fine up until there were some interventions (Pitocin), at which point it became too much for her to handle. One of the nurses mentioned, "I wonder if the baby's head is too large to fit through your pelvis?" At that moment, my friend was taken a direction she did not anticipate. At that time, 1 in 3 babies born in the hospital closest to us turned into a C-section delivery. Typically you can look up the specific C-section rates for your hospital by searching "c-section rates at _____ hospital". Which pulls up a really long list of all the hospitals in America and the percent of births that are C-section deliveries. Our hospital "declined to respond", so I actually called the maternity ward and spoke with the analytics department. Today, the chances are even greater that the birth will end in a C-section. These statistics certainly played a part in my decision to have my baby at home. I watched a documentary called *The Business of Being Born* that was eye-opening as it pertains to this topic. My friend had 6 weeks of recovery after that major surgery. I would say that news made me feel that much more solid in my choice to have a home birth. Research studies on consumerreports.org on *The Danger of Unnecessary C-Sections* show an increase in maternal mortality rates due to complications from this major surgery.

I woke up at 4 a.m. the day before the due date. Let's face it, I woke up at 4 a.m. every morning for the past couple months. That morning though, I see a bear lumbering around in the dumpster. I hear a large metal bang; it's the bear leaving the dumpster after feasting for several hours. I think bears showing up in my life means something. There was also a bear running across the golf course at our wedding six years before this day.

I think due dates are a terrible idea. Especially with the 1st baby. It's all based on the period you most recently had and they count 40 weeks out. Research on *evidencebasedbirth.com* shows with the first baby, its standard for pregnancy to last longer than 40 weeks. In *The Business of Being Born* documentary, they go into how many inductions are performed unnecessarily and that sometimes the baby is really not fully ready to be born. I figured God's design is a good one and that when this baby was ready, the baby would come. I couldn't be pregnant forever, right?

The pressure I placed on myself was immense. I felt it from all directions. I was being regularly adjusted throughout the pregnancy and I honestly have no idea how other pregnant women go without regular chiropractic care. I decided to go get some acupuncture that would help with preparing me for birth. I was getting chiropractic adjustments on a daily basis at this point. Lots of Webster Technique to make sure the baby was going to be in the prime position for birth and my pelvis and low back were aligned. This helped immensely with all of the pregnancy symptoms I was feeling in my low back every day I was on my feet working.

It was the 1st rifle hunting season beginning October 11th. The only way Jacob can go off grid to the ranch to hunt is if I go with. That sounded way better than sitting around waiting for the child to be born. We hopped in the car and headed for the ranch. It was located an hour and a half away. We drove over the mountain pass, which is a bit bumpy but nothing that's too terrible. We began the slow, arduous drive up the ranch road and whoa! Those bumps were so intense that I could not take it at times. I told him he had to stop the car! I'd recover and he'd drive a bit more and I had to have him stop over and over and over again. The pressure on my cervix was more than I could take. I was so sensitive at that point of my pregnancy.

We eventually made it to the cabin and it was 7:15 p.m. I had some soup the hunting party had cooked up and we talked and I went to sleep. Around 11 p.m. I felt some stuff happening. I wasn't sure it was much of anything so I went back to sleep. Around 1 a.m., there was no mistaking it, I was finally in labor!

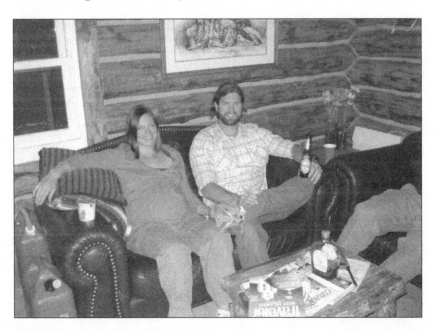

2

GRACE'S
HOME BIRTH

*"Just as a woman's heart knows how and
when to pump, her lungs to inhale, and
her hand to pull back from fire, so she
knows when and how to give birth."*

- VIRGINIA DI ORIO

I'd had the impression labor would feel super intense and unbearable, but it was so mild. Yes, I could feel my entire uterus contract and squeeze for a few minutes and then I'd have a few minutes break. They were regular and increasing to less and less time in between them. Jacob finally came to bed and I told him what was happening. We drove home. Wow, let me tell you, that was a quick ride back to the house. The normally hour-and-a-half car ride felt like it had been cut in half. Jacob was determined to get me home. He was breathing with me as we made our way down the bumpy ranch road and back over Kebler Pass. He was timing the contractions and telling me things like, "You've got this!" and "We are almost home!"

We finally arrived home around 2 a.m. Jacob immediately went into the mode of blowing up the pool and filling it with hot water while I went upstairs to the bed. Annie arrived shortly after we called her and helped me through some contractions. She rubbed me on my back, shoulders and sacrum. She coached me to keep my face relaxed and breathe slowly. The contractions started becoming more and more intense, but still totally okay. I labored in a seated and squatting position upstairs before going downstairs to get into the pool. There was not enough hot water to fill the pool so pots start boiling and they rushed to get it filled so I could get in as soon as possible. It was going pretty well. I drank an enormous carrot juice throughout and ate a fig newton and dried mango and drank Recharge and water as well.

I got into the pool around 4 a.m. and I sat in butterfly pose while Annie pressed downward on my shoulders which felt fabulous. The water was warm and soothing and kept warm with boiling pots of water as well as hot water from the hose attached to the sink. I felt like vomiting around 5 a.m. and Jacob quickly got a bowl and Annie held it near my mouth as I threw up split pea soup (my dinner). I got out of the pool to wash my mouth out and actually felt relief after vomiting. I decided I wanted to lay in bed and rest a while at 5:45 a.m. I didn't sleep much because I went through a contraction every couple minutes. I decided to stand and grab the bedside dresser as I moved my hips back and forth. Jacob was sleeping in the bed and he checked on me every so often. Annie was napping downstairs on the couch. I felt queasy again and went to the bathroom to throw up. Again, I felt relieved. I grabbed the bathroom counter and just went at it, moving my hips all around with every contraction. I reached a point of transition. This is for real, people. It's like the apex of contractions and then you go into this "baby is going to be born soon" mode, and pushing starts. I wanted the birthing pool, but it wasn't ready. Some relief would have been nice right about then! We needed more hot water. I was able to get in the pool shortly after. I remember having had carrot juice at some point. Bad idea. Unless you like having carrot pulp swimming around. It's a bit hard when

11

you start pushing to hold everything in. It really wanted to come out both ends at a certain point.

I was going to town dealing with contractions and pushing. I wondered if it was going to go on forever. It felt like an eternity and I had not slept at all that night. Jacob was so encouraging. Annie was a life saver. Lots of great "just breathe" or "relax your face," etc, and massaging all the right places. I was so out of it that I can't even tell you all the details. I just remember reaching a point of no return. This baby was coming and it was going to happen soon. The contractions seemed back to back and I felt I couldn't relax in between any longer. I let out loud, low yells with each contraction. I kept thinking and saying, "I can't do this." Annie and Jacob kept saying, "You are doing it right now." They were both very encouraging and Annie suggested a change in position, so I got on my knees and spread them wide as I rocked forward and back. I felt like I could not go on much longer. I also felt as if it would never end. Jacob kept bringing more hot water and Annie continued supporting and loving me through it all.

I felt like I was ready to throw in the towel about this time. I got into a deep squat and leaned back into the side of the pool with Jacob on my left and Annie on the right. I felt like pushing a bit with the contractions now. I grabbed both their hands and belted out the loudest, longest yells I could muster. Each contraction went through waves of peaks. During a contraction, I would feel about 4 peaks and yell with each one. I pushed for the last 2-3 peaks of each contraction when I was near the end. I remember saying, "I don't want to have a baby anymore," to which Annie replied, "You don't want to be pregnant forever, right?" That lightened the mood quite well.

Jacob started updating me on the progress I was making with each push. He began by saying the head was only 1" away from exiting the birth canal. Then, he said, "I can see baby's hair," and "Baby is going to come into the world soon." He told me that I needed to push baby out soon. My amniotic sac finally ruptured and a light green/yellow fluid shot out into the pool. Three or 4 contractions later (as the head pushed out and retracted back in several times) the head was so close to being born that Jacob said, "You only have 10% left and the head will be out." So I pushed as hard as I could and felt the most intense, burning and tingling sensation all around my entire vagina, and the baby's head popped out! Jacob felt around the neck for the cord and unwound it from around the baby's neck.

I had a rest in between contractions and with the next contraction her body was out and Jacob began bringing the baby out of the water. She was looking at me when she was under the water. Then, she emerged out of the water. As I held her upright, he suctioned her nose and mouth and she was looking around at me with her big blue eyes. Jacob kept saying, "She's a beautiful baby girl. Honey, you did it!" and "She's so beautiful!" over and over again.

It was like she was born ready to take on the world. So amazing. Her beautiful, clear eyes and face. They were so perfectly shaped and symmetrical. She had such tiny features. I fell in love immediately. The dogs were peeking their heads over the edge of the pool trying to figure out what this new little person was all about. A beam of light shone in from the large window. We'd had our first snow in the early morning. I had done it. I felt exhilarated and happy and unbelievable all at the same time. It was 8:13 a.m.

I was pretty ecstatic at this point and just couldn't take my eyes off of her. Jacob pulled my bra down and I attempted to breastfeed. She latched on a couple times and sucked vigorously for a couple seconds. Jacob phoned family to tell them we had a baby girl while I just sat holding her body against mine, under the water.

The umbilical cord was a beige color and had arteries and veins running through it and it was pulsating. Thirty-five minutes after the birth, Jacob clamped and cut the cord. By then I had a really strong uterine contraction that never let up. Annie helped me through that unexpected tough period of about 30 minutes of my uterus contracting and finally I birthed the placenta in the pool with minimal bleeding. The placenta was enormous, but it did not hurt to squeeze it through my birth canal. All I could feel was the intense uterine contractions. Jacob held our new baby girl throughout the placental birth. He helped lift me out of the pool and then I was freezing and felt quite strange. He robed me and we sat on the couch with our new baby. Jacob brought me soup and Annie took our 1st family photo. I warmed up and thanked Annie profusely for all of her help and truly would not have had the experience I did without her encouragement, touch, breathing assistance, etc.

I did it. In our living room. In a kiddie pool I'd found for $25 that was the perfect size and height. The birth cost us less than $100.

3

NEW MOM

"The moment a child is born,
a mother is born also."

-RAJNEESH

Motherhood. Talk about a 24/7 job, the most rewarding and challenging job of my life.

The newborn stage is incredibly sweet. There was a lot of sleeping. If I were giving myself advice as a new mom, it would be to rest. I know, there's things to do and meals to make and clean up, etc. The cleaning can wait. The food will be provided. Have simple things as far as food is concerned. There's no need to cook anything! Paper plates and plastic utensils for a week, or longer, is not going to hurt anything. I would tell myself that resting and allowing others to support you is priority #1! I say this now because I didn't take adequate time to rest and rejuvenate. Partially due to the fact that I felt so awesome post-birth. Still, allowing my mind and body the time to integrate everything that had just occurred is something I would have liked to give myself more time for.

Immediately following the birth, Annie and Jacob cleaned it all up. I felt weightless and overjoyed, full of energy and empowered beyond belief! I felt like I could do anything! I was invincible! I can remember being with new baby and Madeline, my 7-year-old Lab. Her head was as big as new baby's entire body. I took a picture. I spent a long time staring at this beautiful child that had been in my belly the past 9+ months. It didn't feel real. Eventually, I finally fell asleep that night.

Then the milk came in 2 days later. Up until then, she'd been eating the colostrum (really dense, yellow milk). I was completely engorged and tight like an inflated football. New baby ate like crazy. She loved to nurse. I can still hear her kitten noises to this day, gentle and loving sounds coming from her, so much love pouring through me to her. She had the most perfect features. Symmetrical and defined. Big blue eyes looking at me! I didn't have a breast pump right away, so it was just new baby nursing that finally brought the boobs back to a softer, less football-like feel. My boobs would spray everywhere when the let-down occurred. She's only got one mouth! The other boob didn't seem to care and would also let down and milk would literally spray everywhere. I started wearing boob pads in my bra or placing pressure with my finger on the opposite nipple for a few seconds when starting to feed her. We got it down, her and I. Eventually.

Breast feeding was so powerful. I could feel my uterus contracting back down to its pre-baby size. That 1st week was intense sometimes. It feels like the uterus is clamping down when it's returning to its normal size. I looked like I was still pregnant right after birth. I did gain 20–25 pounds and new baby was 7 lbs 13 1/2 ounces, so I still had a belly there. However, the water weight that comes off in those initial moments following birth is incredible. You're also releasing tons of blood that comes out in clumps. Thank goodness for the pads I'd soaked in witch hazel and stuck in the freezer. Those really helped with the healing down there. The bleeding lasted 6 days for me. It was heavy at first, and decreased to only a bit of bleeding within the first couple days.

I would be doing everyone a disservice if I failed to mention the full healing process down there. A large head is coming out of the vagina. Of course that's traumatic and being my first time, I wasn't sure what to expect. I'm grateful for the witch hazel pads. I also used a funnel to pee. Yep, turned it upside down. When urine touches anything post-birth, it stings like hell. I can remember not wanting to go to the bathroom for fear of the stinging pain I experienced from peeing. Also a great option is a water bottle that you can squirt the area with while peeing. It's a must-have. Before figuring that out, I had to get in the bath tub full of water to go. It works too. Just not what you want to be doing every time you need to go.

It was painful to sit for a few days following birth. I would sit on my foot positioned in a way where there would be absolutely no pressure on my perineal region.

It was time for new baby to have a name! Ten days after her birth we named her Ansley Grace. Named after her Great-Grandma Grace. We called her Grace from the start and she still goes by Grace to this day. There's a lot of meaning in that name. Grandma Grace was a powerful woman, strong and humorous, always laughing and a lovely being. She taught me a lot about enjoying life and I can still hear her distinct laugh that lit up a room!

Getting the birth certificate from the county involved having a notary witness and sign a document signed by 2 witnesses (I chose Annie and my mother) and my doctor (Jacob) that I was indeed pregnant and birthed a child on October 11, 2008 at 8:13 a.m. We then took that to the County Records Office and filled out their paperwork. We did this soon after naming Grace. We wanted to get to know her a bit before naming her. I support everyone in taking your time with this, given that their name is for the rest of their life. A hospital birth requires you to name your child before they release you. That extra time was essential to us in the process of naming our first child.

Co-sleeping: What a beautiful, close and sleepless experience. Need I say more? I don't regret doing it. However, as much as I enjoyed the convenience of not having to get up to feed her in the night, I turned into the all-night snack bar. I became zombie-like and sort of out of touch with reality at times. I was getting such broken sleep. Grace was the typical baby and got up in the night to nurse. Note: There's a large difference between doing that in the beginning stages and also still doing it one and a half years later. Insert horror face emoji here. Talk about losing my mind.

On that note, let me talk about breastfeeding brain. Yeah, it's a thing. More severe for me than pregnancy brain. It's as if all of your brain cells exit through the breast milk. I could barely remember my patients' names that I saw on a weekly basis. Totally normal. Jacob had to repeat things he had just told me. I got glimpses of what it was like before baby, but it felt like it was going to be like this forever. I felt inadequate and wondered how I could not remember all of these things that were so easy pre-baby. It's going to be okay! The memory comes back and you become just as sharp as you were before. It takes time.

All the firsts: She smiles for the first time, words cannot describe the sensations and emotions that flood in. She laughs—precious. She grabs her feet for the first time! She rolls. Crawls. Sits. Stands. Says "Mama" or "Dada." Grace's first word according to her grandfather was "Bapo," so he named himself that when she was 6 months old and he still goes by that today. She runs. She falls asleep in the cutest positions. In her sling, her chair, the bed, the car seat and even the stairs.

She's only a couple weeks old and I'm back at it with the office. I just have her in a sling attached to me at all times. Did I mention how we could only get her to sleep via an up and down motion? Yep, hugging her close and literally doing a squat. She knew the difference between a small drop and a large one. She only slept for the deep squat. I got super great leg workouts. Daily. There's a better way coming later in a book entitled, *Babywise*.

4

PROFESSIONAL LIFE

"The path I took is the right one.
If I had it to do over again, I would do it
over again. Exactly the same way."

-ANONYMOUS

Being a professional and having a new baby is possible. I dedicated an entire chapter to this because I feel it's an important part of my life and I know that many times, a person's career can get in the way of having children or vice versa. I'm a driven person by nature, however, I know many men and women who have a baby and become even more motivated to succeed and provide. With conceiving Grace and starting our business simultaneously, we were taking the leap in all regards. We dove all in. Ready to do whatever it took to make it work in as smooth and effortless a way as possible. Given that I felt so amazing immediately after birth, I got right back into being a chiropractor, working side by side with my husband while Grace was in the baby sling. She was constantly attached to me or her daddy.

There were little if any times she was not in contact with us—unless our patients were holding her. She was in the office whenever we were. There were many benefits to having her there, as well as some challenges.

I encourage you to discover what works best for your situation. This is my experience and what worked for our family. It may look completely different for you. The main thing here, is that it *is* possible and you can do it!

The priority was to keep our family together and close, and we successfully accomplished that. Your priority may differ from ours, and that's okay. Grace was in the office full-time for the first couple years. She would breastfeed when she needed to breastfeed, sleep when she needed to sleep and get changed when she needed changing. I remember altering our hours to fit her nap schedule. Not everyone can do this, nevertheless, it's one example of many things that are conducive to having a baby and a business at the same time. People totally get it, depending on what line of work you're in. Sometimes she and I would be home because of whatever reason and all the patients would ask about her and were almost upset about her not being in the office. It's interesting how that works. Here we thought it was an inconvenience, when really it's something they looked forward to.

I really had to get over the fact that she screamed. A lot. In the office, at home or wherever we went. It's hard when it's your first and you're trying to look picture perfect and like everything's so easy. Let's be real, it's not. And people get it. They understand. Especially if they've got kids. If they do not understand, that's alright too. I decided not to let other people dictate my life. There's a point where you have enough to think about with just you and your baby, and you don't need to fill your plate with worrying about other people. Take care of you and your baby's needs first.

Grace's presence actually catapulted the practice and got us to greater levels. In a way, I feel like babies are magnets! Everyone loves them. We found this to be true with our subsequent children as well.

5

AGAIN!
BREASTFEEDING
AND PREGNANT

*"For you created my inmost being; you knit me
together in my mother's womb. I praise you
because I am fearfully and wonderfully made;
your works are wonderful, I know that full well."*

- PSALM 139:13-14

I was breastfeeding Grace on a regular basis. She was eighteen months old and I really got the feeling that I wanted to have another. To be able to put into words what that felt like exactly is difficult. It was a strong yearning, a sense of longing. Longing for that beautiful human being. It was a feeling of living into my fullest potential as a woman. I do remember, after Grace was born, I thought that I may not want to do it again. So there I was and I really, really wanted to do it again! I decided that because my period had started up again that it would probably be possible to get pregnant. So we began trying quite regularly. I had a general idea of when my ovulation day was but wasn't 100% certain because it was sporadic at this point. It had been over 2 years since I had had my last period. Things were still integrating and getting back into the flow of my natural cycle.

A couple months passed by with no success. I decided to cut back to two feedings; first thing in the morning and one at night. That did the trick! Finally, after doing it daily for what felt like forever (two or three months), I was pregnant! I took the test thinking there was no way it would be positive. I hadn't had a period in four weeks, so I figured I'd rule out pregnancy. I was elated! Baby #2! I told Jacob and he was sad he wasn't there for the pregnancy test itself. This is the second time this had happened now. What can you do? Again, I had thought it would be negative.

My pregnancy, along with breastfeeding Grace was starting to take its toll on me. I felt drained all the time. Literally and figuratively. Two or three months into the pregnancy, when Grace was two years old, I weaned her completely. It was bittersweet. I had to go with my gut here.

Things began to feel way better with my pregnancy and my life in general. Our practice was booming. We were traveling every two months for conferences in Atlanta. Traveling with Grace was an adventure. She screamed a lot. We got our workout in every time we were on the plane with her. Eventually it got to the point where I left Grace with my folks because it was getting to be too much. She was weaned now and I was becoming quite pregnant. We actually decided to begin driving from Crested Butte to the neighboring town every Tuesday and Thursday morning to accommodate our practice members from the other town. This is a thirty-minute commute one way. We had to wake up quite early in order to be there by 8 a.m. That was a challenging time for me. I am not a morning person, and during pregnancy, I require quite a bit more sleep. I made it happen. Jacob and I were a great team. We did what we needed to do to make things really grow within our business.

This eventually included looking into buying a home. We looked all over our region for years to no avail. Then, when I was searching the neighboring town one day, I discovered a new listing. It only had a description and a picture of the front of the house. I knew this was the one. It was 3 bed/2 bath/2-car garage with a little yard. Perfect! Up until then, we had been looking at dumps and were pretty much over it. We immediately went to look at it and we bought it. The mortgage application process was intense. Especially being we had hundreds of thousands in student loan debt. They do a ratio that shows your liabilities compared to your assets. Ours was on the "we have way more debt than assets" end of things. They do not make it easy even if your income is amazing. We were barely able to qualify. It was approved and I spent the next month or so preparing for the move.

I feel like it's important to note that I was walking and hiking regularly as well as eating at Ryce weekly. The drunken noodle bowl with tofu was something I regularly had cravings for. One of the benefits of living in a high-end tourist town is good food! Another thing that's important for my health is being vegan. At this point, I'd been vegan eight years. You can be vegan and produce really healthy babies and breastfeed those babies! I enjoyed fresh vegetable juices throughout my pregnancies and it really helped me get in my greens. All the vitamins and minerals needed can be provided by a vegan diet. I took a vegan pre-natal as well. There were some days I craved salads and others all I wanted was lots and lots of carbohydrates or protein-rich vegan foods.

I was also chasing around a toddler. Grace was into everything. One day she decided to rub diaper cream all over her body and douse herself with powder. She was completely white, even her face. That child was and still is very spirited. This classification came from a book I read called *Secrets of the Baby Whisperer*, which I read in hopes of getting Grace to sleep better.

I noticed I was feeling really good, overall, with my pregnancy. Sometimes, I felt like I was starving, but didn't want to eat anything. If you've been pregnant before, I think you'll be able to relate to that. At one of the conferences we attended, I felt extremely nauseated and couldn't throw up. Our mentor at the time, a great chiropractor, adjusted me and I immediately vomited and I felt a lot better. Other than those things, I actually felt better pregnant than not.

In my journal, I noted Braxton-Hicks contractions 2 months before her birth. I hadn't had those until 1 month before the birth of Grace. My body seemed to know more the 2nd time around. Sleep was becoming uncomfortable around that time as well. New baby was making slow, large movements more often. I also journaled about how I was falling in love with new baby more and more with every passing day. The bonding experience for me began well before birth.

Everything was coming together at once: new house, new baby, new office! We'd outgrown our office space and moved to a much larger space. It required a build-out that Jacob was very skilled at doing. He built some of the rooms and the entire front counter that encompassed all of the electrical as well. We were there for one another through this enormous growth phase. The support I felt from him in my pregnancy was helpful. I could tell he really cared about my wellbeing. He wouldn't even let me lift a finger in the build-out.

In March, I began packing up the place in preparation for our move. I was waking constantly around 3 in the morning, feeling energized and ready to go! About this time, Grace was completely potty-trained. She responded very well to gummy vitamins, which I gave her every time she went on the toilet. She even quit wearing diapers at night. The process was very smooth. I most definitely took that for granted. She just had this innate drive. She's a very determined child.

My ideal scene for the birth of our second child was this:

Labor in a relaxed atmosphere at home with freedom to be in any and all rooms. Warm with heat source being the wood-burning stove. Birthing pool in the living room with kitchen sink as main hot water source. Boiling pots of water ready to go as well. Grace there. Bring Annie over once contractions become unbearable. Jacob could set up entire water birth in 1 hour. Wait to fill pool until well into birth. Have lots of Recharge, tea and juice on hand. Babysitters were on standby if Grace got overwhelmed. Blinds/shades drawn. Candles would be nice. No noise. Lots of towels. Bathrobes as well. Fully clothed before birthing pool. Bathing suit top on for birth. No video. Pictures okay. Breathe throughout and listen to Annie's relaxation cues. Change positions frequently. More physical contact with Jacob. Hugging. Resting while hugging his neck in a semi-squat position. Think "open." Let go. Don't struggle. Let the baby just come out. No holding back. It was helpful for me to think about these things in advance, and I went over it with Annie and Jacob.

On March 19th, I recorded having had regular, consistent Braxton-Hicks contractions during the previous two nights. I also noted that I wanted to be completely moved into the new house before baby came.

Grace was really anticipating new baby and said she wanted both a brother *and* a sister! At this point, I had just learned of the *On Becoming Babywise* book and I was making notes that I needed to read it! I wanted a different sleeping experience the second time around. The whole family needed to be getting good sleep. *Babywise* makes a claim that your baby will sleep through the night by 9 weeks old. I didn't believe it was even possible after what we'd experienced with Grace.

I was talking to Jacob about Grace being in the house during the birth, and that if she watched, that would be fine with me. I showed her videos on YouTube of other home births and she was super excited. I thought to myself how valuable that would have been had I been able to witness a birth, in its natural form, before I went through it myself. I believe that there's so much fear surrounding birth. I certainly never saw anything but screaming and pain when it came to what was on TV. Birth is such a beautiful thing. I feel like being exposed to birth is empowering. It shows how strong and capable a woman is. It was described to me as a child as something that "can" be done naturally. My mom talked about her experience with it. My parents made a huge effort to have natural births. That was not easy back in the 80s. The closest midwife to them was an hour and a half away. They were committed though. I was the firstborn and my mom also had regular chiropractic care leading up to all of our births. After only five hours of labor, I came into the world. My mom is a strong woman. When she sets her mind to something, she does it! And my dad is the most supportive person I know, always approaching life with a can-do attitude. He had to drive fast and was pulled over by the police on the way to the hospital.

I am grateful to have had natural birth modeled for me. Growing up in a household where that was normal definitely helped me. Saying all that, I do have many friends that go natural with their births where the opposite was modeled to them. The pattern can be changed. Ultimately, I believe that many more women are making the choice to go with the innate instincts of giving birth naturally and I see it becoming the new normal soon.

On March 29th, we moved out of our condo. With all the helpers we had, it only took 1 hour to get moved out and 2 hours to get moved in. My packing and organization ahead of time paid off!

On April 1st, my journal says that I had Braxton-Hicks contractions the entire night. Not painful at all, just tiring and annoying. They were coming on every 7 minutes and lasting about 1 minute.

I kept writing about how blessed I felt with the house and my upcoming birth—thanking God. The new house smell was pretty extreme to me with my sense being so heightened. Annie told me that citrus would help soak it up, so I placed large bowls of lemons and oranges in the house to absorb the construction chemical smells. Our mattress was on the floor and it was getting more and more difficult to get up and go to the bathroom in the night.

On April 15th, I noted that new baby was up to something! I checked my cervix and realized I was two centimeters dilated. This was me simply putting two fingers inside my vagina and feeling up into my cervix. You'll feel a cone-like object if you try this. Feel inside the tip of the cone and you can tell if you're dilated because your fingers can go inside of the tip of the cone (cervix). If you aren't dilated, the tip of the cervix will be closed and you can't put a finger deep inside of it.

I was going through some interesting feelings. Up until that day, I was observing baby and could tell that the head was down. Today, felt like something completely different. I also noted that a full moon was coming up soon. I had read that babies are more likely to be born on or near a full moon. Everything was ready to go as far as the birthing pool (the kiddie pool) and birthing supplies.

April 18th: Baby dropped! It occurred after a long walk. I could not handle any negativity whatsoever at this point in my pregnancy. I was ready to embrace new baby and the experience was going to be wonderful.

The final picture of me before the birth of baby #2!

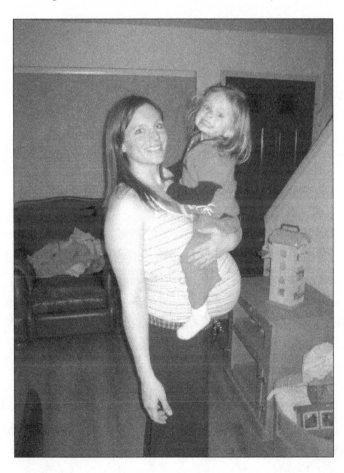

6

ADA'S HOME BIRTH

*"Birth is not only about making babies.
Birth is about making mothers—strong,
competent, capable mothers who trust
themselves and know their inner strength."*

- BARBARA KATZ ROTHMAN

I began labor 9:45 p.m. on the actual due date, April 20th, 2011. I wasn't positive it was true labor because I'd had similar, painless contractions weeks and days before. I was both hoping for labor and not wanting to go into labor all at the same time. I wanted to go into labor and meet this baby and I also felt like going to sleep for the night would be nice as well. I felt this anticipation of what was about to happen. Like many times in life, the anticipation can be more intense than the very thing we are anticipating.

At 12:50 a.m. I texted Annie and told her I was definitely in labor and to please come. I felt most comfortable standing in our bathroom with both hands on the counter. I would move my hips forward with every contraction and squeeze my arms alongside my belly and breathe out long, deep "oh" or "ah" sounds. I did about 4 deep breaths per contraction. My eyes were closed from this time on. I visualized my cervix going from cone shaped and small to spreading out and forming an enormous opening for the baby's head to slip right out. I did not think about doing this prior to birth. In fact, the first time the thought entered my mind was in the midst of labor.

Jacob set up the birthing pool in the bedroom and filled it while I labored in the bathroom. Annie arrived at 1 a.m. and immediately came in and began putting downward pressure on my shoulders. It felt much better during contractions. She also breathed with me and spoke out "open" and "out" while I was going through contractions. I had some large bowel movements and peed during this time and it helped. While in the bathroom, I really felt the urge to push several times. I transitioned onto the bed next and relaxed in a child's pose type position with a pillow during breaks.

After the bed, I transitioned to the birth pool and had a lengthy period of rest followed by several contractions all in a row with little to no breaks. I chose an all fours position and rocked forward and back. The contractions were all bearable, but I felt like they would never end. All of a sudden I had that irresistible pushing urge, which surprised me, and I went at it. My water broke and Jacob came into the room at that point and said I was only 10 contractions away from birthing new baby. I felt the head was close. I pushed with every contraction and felt very open. I no longer felt that cramping pain in my cervix. Three contractions later, the head was bulging and I put my hand down there to put pressure on the head as it felt like it would explode out. Jacob also put his hands on her head and helped with the counter pressure.

The head was born and I couldn't believe it. No pain whatsoever. I'd read about this and thought those women were either crazy or lying. And here I was, feeling all warm and fuzzy about what had just happened. That was a different experience than the ring of fire I'd felt with Grace. Once the head was out, it was only seconds until the body slipped out and Jacob unraveled the cord from around new baby's neck and she came out of the water into my arms. He saw we'd had a girl! Her eyes stayed shut and barely opened. There was this very grumpy look on her face. She was so mellow. She stretched out a couple times in the water and then acted as if she was still in the womb. She did not want to open her eyes at all. She took her first breaths. I remember feeling so grateful and thanking God for this precious baby girl.

Jacob suctioned fluid out of her nose and mouth. Annie took photos and video. Ada Jane was born at 3:45 a.m., April 21, 2011. She was beautiful. She didn't make a peep. The cord stopped pulsating around 20 minutes post birth. Jacob cut it and put a cord ring on. The placenta came 1 hour and 15 minutes post birth with the aid of Ada nursing. I felt fabulous! Thank you God for a healthy baby girl! And thank God for regular chiropractic care leading to a quick and speedy delivery! We checked and adjusted her. She had an immediate response and her entire body felt more relaxed. At 9 a.m. she ate for 40 minutes and was easy to latch on. Not much mess or clean up to do. Jacob emptied and deflated pool. We had a morning nap with all four of us on the bed.

It was lovely.

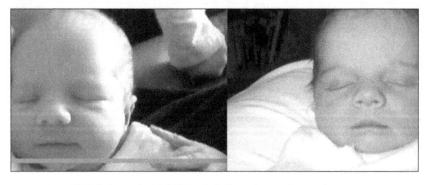

A side by side of Ada's and Grace's newborn photos.

7

BABYWISE: SLEEP IS GOOOOD

"Rest and be thankful."

- WILLIAM WADSWORTH

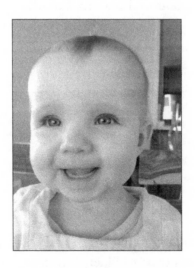

Maybe the most important chapter yet! The first thing I need to say is read the book, *On Becoming Babywise* by Gary Ezzo M.A. & Robert Bucknam M.D. Yes, it looks super outdated and it was written a loooooong time ago. The information is relevant and it works. They make claims that your baby will be sleeping through the night by 7 to 9 weeks old, and you won't be doing the cry it out method in order to achieve this. This has been reproduced by thousands of people over and over again. They show consistent results on babies with all sorts of backgrounds, personalities and dispositions.

My pastor gave me this book. His daughter had utilized the Babywise principles for her kids and told me all about how simple it was and that it really worked. In the late stages of my pregnancy with Ada, I had decided to read it. Some of it seemed so simple that I thought to myself, "How does this actually work?" I had my doubts about it working for our children. I thought that we must simply produce kids that can't sleep through the night. Grace was a co-sleeper, and I felt like her all-night snack bar. She seemed to eat more at night than during the day. It was difficult to imagine this simple routine working for us. One of the first things they talk about is sleeping the baby in a separate room after 10 days old.

Firstly, they recommend making sure the baby is getting a *full* feeding every time you breastfeed them. So, when the baby instantly nods off upon beginning to feed them, you basically need to keep them awake so they're eating as much as possible for as long as possible.

Secondly, you need to keep in mind this order of things after the baby is 10 days old:

1st-Feed
2nd-Awake/Play time (in the beginning this is extremely short)
3rd-Sleep

The cycle starts off around 2-2 1/2 hours long and increases to 3-3 1/2 hours long as they get older. The most important part of the cycle is that you are *not* feeding your baby before they nap. You are not using feeding to get them to fall asleep. Unless it's right before night sleeping (bedtime). Feed, awake, sleep. Repeat. That's it! Before nighttime sleep, you feed them as much as possible before laying them down for the night.

The premise behind the method is that it works with the metabolism and the body's sleep cycle. Metabolism affects the length and quality of sleep. If the digestive system is constantly having to work, it interferes with the length of sleep. This cycle where the baby is only eating when they wake up from sleeping sets them up for longer stretches of sleep at night. It's genius!

I had Ada and immediately implemented the getting as full a feeding as possible. At 10 days old, she moved into a bassinet in her own room. Part of the reason for this is because they can't smell you and won't be as likely to wake up as frequently in the night. From 10 days old through 6 1/2 weeks, she would get up about 1-2 times in the night to eat and immediately go back to sleep. By 6 1/2 weeks old, she was sleeping 8 hours or more every single night! I was amazed.

How do you get them to fall asleep, you might ask? This part was intimidating to me in the beginning. Another key to Babywise is the baby being able to self-soothe, meaning they don't need rocking, vibration, bouncing or other lengthy sleep routines in order to fall asleep. You literally lay the baby down when there's been sufficient awake time and they're yawning or rubbing their eyes, and you leave the room. I made sure it was dark and comfortable. You don't make a big thing of it. The first few times you do this, there may be some crying. If it lasts more than 5-10 minutes, go in and check the baby and comfort them. Then you leave the room again. They will likely go to sleep within 1 to 2 cycles of this. Eventually, they go to sleep within a minute or two. Ada took to this after a couple times. After that, I just laid her down and there was zero crying and she put herself to bed. Clearly, if your baby is sick or not well, you'll need to alter things during that period of time. It's important to be there for your baby when they really need you.

We got to the point where sleeping was fun! I was getting lots of sleep, and Ada was regularly sleeping 13 hours straight at night. I pumped sometimes to make sure I wouldn't have a clogged milk duct.

It's nice to begin storing milk in the freezer for the future. Lavender essential oil is awesome for helping to prevent clogged milk ducts, mixed with any carrier oil like coconut or almond oil. Rub all over the boob. I never had mastitis or any side effects of going long periods without breastfeeding her at night. I had experienced mastitis when breastfeeding Grace. It may have occurred because I had slept on my belly a couple times and that clogged the milk ducts on one side. However, given the amount of feedings throughout the night, it's wild that anything could have become clogged.

Ada was a very happy baby and all of us were happy because we were getting great sleep! Bedtime was easy. Naps were treasured and protected. Maybe overly so. They can nap on the go as well. My babies always slept longer at home. When on a cycle like this, they eat a lot when it's eat time! I had to make sure I was getting enough calories throughout my day. I felt the complete opposite with Ada compared to how I felt with Grace as far as being rested. Do I regret the way we did it with Grace? No. The co-sleeping was a nice bonding experience, but I felt like a zombie for 18 months. I definitely learned a lot from that experience. If my story isn't convincing enough, please read the *Babywise* book. It talks about all the nitty gritty details concerning all the possibilities when implementing the technique. It really is as simple as making sure you stick to the order of feed, awake, sleep.

Another aspect of *Babywise* is that as baby gets bigger and eventually eats solid food along with milk feedings, the cycle length gets longer. More towards the 3 1/2 hour mark for one feed, awake, nap cycle. Sometimes they nap the majority of the cycle! It's like that during the newborn stage. I will say, every baby is extremely different with when they want solids. Grace was 13 months old before she'd eat solids, whereas Ada took to solids at 7 months old. That also coordinated with when they each got their first tooth!

After not sleeping through the night for 18 months post Grace's birth, I was open to trying just about anything. I'm glad I didn't go with something complicated or unrealistic. This is a method that is a winning situation for all involved! No more sleep-deprivation and spending hours trying to get your baby to sleep. I remember doing squats for a minimum of 15 minutes to get Grace to sleep. It was a workout! It is unbelievable the lengths we went to in order to get her to sleep. I know there are so many gadgets out there for sleep—special vibrating beds and rocking and swings and noise makers, etc. The list is infinite. You do not need to buy anything to get your baby to sleep. As long as they have the comforts of a nice, cozy bed and a dark room, you are good to go.

I tell all of my patients about this book, as well as my friends and family. I have spoken with a baby sleep therapist that teaches this method to her clients. I do not know of a better method.

Thank you, *Babywise*!

8

THE GIRLS

"My life, my love, my heart, my children."

- ANONYMOUS

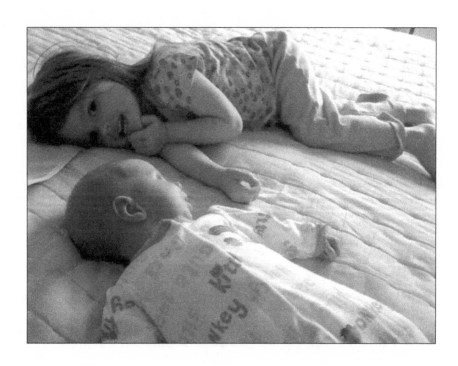

Now that you know I was actually getting plenty of rest and Ada was sleeping really well, let's get into the experience of having a newborn along with a toddler. It really is a whirlwind of an adventure. Grace had a big sister party shortly after Ada's birth where she got presents and a cake. It went a long way for making her feel special. This reminds me of Madeline, my first dog. I got her at the beginning of college when I was in a 1-bedroom apartment. She was my companion. Then many transitions took place that she had to get used to. I got married, then we adopted another dog and had kids. She certainly felt demoted on several of those transitions. Grace's experience of having a new baby sister was the opposite of that. She knew she played an enormous role in the family dynamic and she took to that with helping, even if it only involved bringing me diapers or playing with Ada while I was busy with other things.

I felt so amazing after my home water birth with Ada that I got right back into the office within a few weeks. She was with me and I nursed and napped her in the office for a while before transitioning into a pattern of having a babysitter bring her to me to nurse when she woke from her nap. My schedule was such that I had time with the girls in the morning, a couple hours in the afternoon and then I was home in the late evening. My work hours were 11-1 and 3-7 with Ada breastfeeding when I was home and at some point during the evening shift. It took some getting used to. I remember feeling really great about the way things were going between home life and work life. I liked having both.

Working alongside my husband was fun. We synergized well. Not to say we didn't have some challenging times as well, in the form of disagreements or needing to work through stuff. When we focused on our strengths and supporting one another, things went a lot better.

Ada was tiny when she was born, just under 6 pounds. She put on weight quickly and was a great eater. With the motivation from *Babywise*, I really focused on her getting in those full feedings, and it worked! She went from 6 pounds all the way up to 7 pounds in 1 week.

She continued to chunk up and her cheeks got really big and cute. Grace was helpful at times like I mentioned earlier, with bringing me diapers when I needed more or entertaining Ada when she was fussing and I couldn't get to her immediately. Ada rarely fussed. Grace cried more than Ada at this point and required more attention and entertainment. It's interesting how that worked out. In a way, it was easier having two than it was with just one kid.

Grace was finally in her big girl bed in her own room when we moved into our first home. She was so excited to hold her new baby sister for the first time. At 2 1/2, she was pretty distracted and getting into a lot of things. She was kind of in a "no" stage. She hated hearing the word no. I think we were going through some terrible 2's where listening was difficult and I was very busy. Making a mess was really easy for her to do. She was hilarious at times. I remember her always doing something, whether it be riding the dogs, going to the ranch with Daddy, coloring, creating things, getting into lotions and potions, not napping, attempting to play with Ada (Ada just laid there so sweetly), lots and lots of screaming while trying to get her to sleep at night or getting into trouble. She'd come to the office here and there, not every day like it had been in the past.

I went for frequent walks with the girls, putting them in the chariot. We even took bike rides. With the infant sling attachment for the stroller, they were both comfortable riding inside during spring, summer, fall or winter. I even stuck Ada in the ergo baby carrier for hikes here and there and Jacob would have Grace in a backpack. We were an active family.

We traveled quite a bit for conferences that Jacob and I spoke at across the country. Grace started to have one-on-one time with her grandparents for these conferences. Ada came with us so I could breastfeed. She was a good traveler, very content and happy. It was so nice to be sleeping through the night. Ada's first trip occurred when she was about 4 weeks old. Although she wasn't sleeping through the night by then, it was doable to get up and feed her once during the night within the close quarters of a hotel room.

DR. LAURA SIMS D.C.

Grace and Ada continued to blossom and their personalities really shone through. Grace was fiery and driven. Ada was angelic and smiled all the time. Ada truly had the sweetest disposition—partly her personality and also because she was getting a lot of sleep! I recall her going to bed at 8 p.m. and sleeping until 9 a.m. the majority of the time. I had to wake her up to feed her at 9 a.m. Who knows, she may have slept even longer had I not! I had an entire nursing and diaper set-up in her bedroom nightstand as well as my nightstand in my bedroom. It was super handy for dealing with burping and leaking milk as well as changing her after feedings. I remember having to shake her to keep her awake or use a wet washcloth to get her to eat as much as possible. Frequent jiggling took place. She endured a lot of annoying things in order to stay awake! I'm so grateful for both my girls. They did well together and the 2 1/2-year age difference seemed to work well.

Ada took to eating solids at 7 months. She started with bananas and avocados. She liked the banana baby food pouches. Pouches weren't around for Grace, so this was a big deal! Ada still breastfed and would eat solids afterward. She was the sweetest and cleanest eater. She also had amazing hand-eye coordination with that spoon!

We had lots of visitors and regular opportunities to go to the ranch, just an hour and a half away. Summers out here are so beautiful. Life was good: new house and new office space that was perfect for accommodating our growth. With Ada's birth, came huge growth! We were seeing hundreds of patients per week near the end of my pregnancy with her, and it doubled within the next 2 years.

No matter your dreams and goals in life, just know, you can do anything. Looking back, it's some of the best memories of my life. Including the girls in the office as well as having time with them at home, we built our hours around our family's needs as well as our patients' needs. Yes, we worked late, but we also had lots of quality family time in the mornings. Mid-afternoon nap times were so helpful. We took the time to enjoy them when they were small and so precious. You can design your life to be anything you want. It is a choice. It was a lot of work to get the perfect situation with work and family balance. The energy you direct towards your dreams, when done in a hyper-focused manner, pays off big time in the end. There were plenty of experiences with the little girls in the office screaming that felt really hard. I know others that bring help with them to the office or have family helping, which we definitely did as well. For the most part, we did it for a long time with just us. I'm really grateful for family and external help, and these things are necessary during certain seasons.

9

CYCLE TRACKING FOR GETTING PREGNANT OR NATURAL BIRTH CONTROL

"The journey is the destination."

-DAN ELDON

I have learned so much over the past several years when it comes to the timing of my period, ovulation and all the sensations with becoming pregnant. There are several methods for tracking your cycle and I will be talking about the ones that I've tried and my experiences with them.

It began with the Lady Comp. This is a device that has a thermometer attached for you to take your basal body temperature first thing in the morning before you get out of bed. It has a place for you to record when you're on your period, and also gives specifics on when you'll be ovulating and when your period will begin next cycle, etc. I used this for years and really liked the ease of it. There wasn't a lot to it. My device broke a couple of times and after the 2nd time, I decided to try a free app called Ovia.

For the Ovia app, I had the luxury of adding several months of data in regard to my past periods and ovulation. However, you can start from scratch with it. It will take a few months to figure your cycle out, at which point it will work just as well for you as it did for me. It was way more interactive and had me input how I was feeling, if I was having a period, how much sleep I was getting, my temperature from first thing in the morning (I kept a thermometer on my bed side table), activity level, nutrition, cervical mucus, location of my cervix (low, middle, high), cervix feeling open or closed, intercourse, pregnancy tests, ovulation tests, and much more. I found this to be more informative and helpful to look back on. Also, there's an Ovia Pregnancy app for when you conceive that takes you from finding out your pregnant all the way through birth and gives tons of information every day about the development of your baby.

When attempting to get pregnant, this simplified the process so much. You know your 6-day fertile window and exactly what days those are. You also know ovulation day. Your temperature rises, ever so slightly, the day you ovulate. I really like knowing where I'm at throughout the month. I learned that my cycle is only 24 days total. The average woman's cycle is 28-30 days. There's something about knowing that your period is about to begin and exactly what day it will start. So helpful! There are days you may feel up or down or all over the place with your mood, and the Ovia app talks about how you may be feeling at certain times throughout your cycle. Resting during certain periods of time is crucial to a woman's body rhythms. Listening to your body and your inner knowing. I find it supportive to know that whatever I experience throughout my cycle is normal and completely understandable.

I felt it when implantation occurred with my 4th pregnancy. It was a new sensation to me. I wasn't as in tune with my body when it came to getting pregnant the first 3 times. The hormones released in my body after implantation and I felt a full uterus when the placenta and embryo were connecting into my blood supply. It's intense and so beautiful. Our bodies are amazing.

Honing into our bodies' natural rhythms is empowering. It's something I plan to tell my girls about before they begin menstruating. I think every girl needs to know how her body works and what to expect. It's how God designed our bodies and it serves an important purpose. It's a great feeling when you already know, going into your period, exactly what's going to happen and that it's normal and healthy. It's also important when it comes to getting pregnant. It takes the guesswork out of it completely.

Lady Comp vs. Ovia app: They both are excellent at letting you know when you'll be ovulating. Lady Comp costs $400-$450 whereas the Ovia app is free. Lady Comp takes the guesswork out of everything. You simply hear the alarm to take your temp first thing in the morning and it does the rest. Ovia app goes into way more detail and you can log so much more information. They both take some time to really get your cycle down pat. I remember when I first began using the Lady Comp it took 4 months before it started telling me the information I began using it for in the first place. It was completely worth it ultimately. The Ovia app requires you to be really on it with entering information every day. Consistency is key!

Fun fact: If you have sex in your fertile zone in the days prior to ovulation, it increases the chances that you will have a girl. Sex on ovulation day or the day after that increases the chances of having a boy. The reason for this is that boy sperm are faster than girl sperm, but the boy sperm doesn't live as long as girl sperm. So if you have sex the day of ovulation (when the egg is released into the fallopian tube), the boy sperm are more likely to reach the egg before the girl sperm. Sex in the days prior to ovulation, increases the chances of a girl sperm penetrating the egg first because they live longer in the uterus. If anything, this would make for a fun experiment. And obviously, we hadn't done this experiment, yet.

10

OVERDUE -
44 WEEKS

"God has perfect timing; never early, never late. It takes a little patience and it takes a lot of faith but it's worth the wait."

-ANONYMOUS

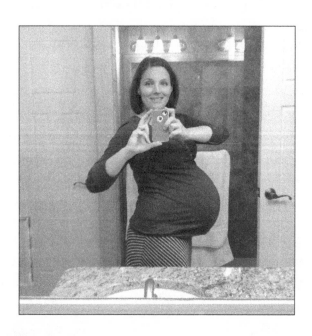

W e decided it was time for #3. August of 2014, I found out I was pregnant. It didn't take long. I guess we got it on the first go. I had a way better idea of where I was in my cycle thanks to the Lady Comp. It made it easy. I had bought some ovulation tests you pee on, but got pregnant before getting a chance to use them. That's divine timing. We were so excited. I approached this pregnancy with enthusiasm and excitement. Preparing lists of what exactly I wanted or needed for the birth. I did so much planning as to what I was eating and getting all the nutrients needed—lots of raw fruits and vegetables along with healthy grains and juicing. Jacob was the best at making me juice and being supportive with my eating and taking care of myself throughout.

At 8 weeks along I wrote that I was feeling puffy and my boobs had doubled in size. Ouch. I was having bouts of hunger that led to some higher calorie days, but definitely not every day. I listened to my body and ate intuitively most of the time. I was extremely active with jogging and took lots of good hikes. I felt pretty amazing. I did note that I had a strange feeling I couldn't describe. Not an aversion and not nausea. Just different.

Keeping a gratitude journal helped along the way. I noted new baby and my family and the abundance in my life, as well as the beginnings of simplified living. I wrote about my health, my bed, our vehicles, our home, helping people, warmth, proper protection, etc.

I craved cooked foods a lot more. I would still have a raw breakfast and lunch, but ended up eating cooked meals at dinner.

I went on a trip to Canada over Labor Day weekend to see my Grandma and my mom's side of the family. Apparently being pregnant does not exempt you from the explosives detection trace portal, or what I refer to as the "puffer" machine. I made it to where they lived in Ontario. My Grandma Grace was dying of lung cancer. I visited with her and it was difficult because she didn't look like my Grandma anymore. Her hair was sparse and she looked gaunt. Her eyes were present though. She was completely herself in personality. She was still laughing and doing whatever she wanted when people would try to get her to eat or drink and she had zero appetite. She told them "I'm not eating that!" in a matter of fact, yet very comical, way. It was challenging to see her like this, and I remember thinking that she'd never get to meet this baby inside of me. I felt mixed emotions. Because while my Grandmas spirit was in the process of departing this earth, a new one would be entering shortly thereafter.

My appetite was up and down and I wrote *a lot* about ideas of foods I might have actually enjoyed eating. Then, when I got them home from the store, I no longer wanted to eat them!

At 13 weeks I wrote that it felt like the pregnancy was going to last forever and that no food was desirable to me. I wrote a list of things that were working for me:

1. Vegan. High raw fruits & greens
2. Consistent exercise 3X/week
3. No oil
4. No salt
5. Home food prep rather than going out
6. 9 hours or more sleep at night

October included Graces 6th birthday party and hot springs! Grace hugged new baby several times and Ada would tickle my belly and say, "I'm tickling the baby!" I began feeling fluttering at 12 weeks pregnant and more definitive movements at 14 weeks.

At the end of October, we went to a chiropractic conference Jacob was speaking at and when he dropped us at the front with all the bags, I overdid it. I carried them all to the room with no help and I started to bleed. I freaked out about it and immediately took a bath and rested. I bled a bit more that night and into the next day. It was very light bleeding. This was a first for me. I was almost 3 months along. I never had anything like that happen the remainder of the pregnancy. I spoke with a colleague who had a similar experience with one of her pregnancies. It was helpful to speak with some one I trusted about what I was going through and she really helped to set my mind at ease about it.

On the topic of work, I was still very involved with the office and marketing events which involved health screenings for the community. It was taxing on me to stand during marketing events which were about 4-5 hours long. I began phasing out of the marketing but remained full-time in the office.

With my exercise routine I was regularly walking and jogging with a good friend. It was incredibly supportive to my self-care and pregnancy.

Thanksgiving was beautiful. We had both our parents and friends and family there. It was so amazing to be together like that—at our kitchen table plus an extra table to for all 12 of us. It stands out as one of my favorite Thanksgivings ever.

My Grandma Grace passed away Christmas Day. I cried. A lot of emotions came up in me and I allowed the full extent of them to wash over me and through me and out of me. It was mixed with gratitude and remembering all of the joy and laughter that she had exuded. It got me thinking about what was really important, and it began a new chapter in my life with how I approached stuff. I mean physical stuff at this point.

I started a capsule wardrobe! The minimalist capsule wardrobe represents the simple core of clothing that you can wear each day and every season. Creating a minimalist capsule wardrobe can simplify your life to the point that you can concentrate on more important things going on and those things you enjoy doing. I also created a dream post-pregnancy capsule wardrobe. It made getting dressed far simpler. I had about 37 pieces. Many of the pieces went together and could mix and match.

I wrote a list of things we'd done right and according to our belief system and I encourage you all to do the same.

Here's my list of things that are in alignment with my values and beliefs that I've (we've) fully embraced:

- Chiropractic
- Home births
- No vaccines
- Home school
- Debt free
- Live in a small mountain town in a great location
- Great work ethic
- Mostly organic diet
- No TV
- Financial goals met
- Focus on being with family
- Food stores—large supply in the event of an emergency
- Garden
- Vehicles paid for
- Fluoride free water
- Lots of smoothies and juicing
- Surround ourselves with a good network
- God
- Minimal
- Good systems and procedures in business
- High morals and values
- Great home
- Great health
- Easy access to skiing, fishing, hiking, sledding, rafting, walking, skating, swimming, hunting
- Lots of time spent with girls
- Not a lot of excess stuff
- Contributions/Giving/Blessing People

What I learned from this pregnancy:

- Patience
- Drive
- Persistence
- Love
- Perseverance
- Importance of support
- Family closeness
- Emotion
- It's okay to feel huge and be huge
- More compassion
- Less is more
- Consumerism is a lie
- Building relationships is more important
- Gratitude
- Less stuff=Less cleaning
- Raw produce is the bomb
- Salt is powerful
- Babies move a lot!
- Cherish the small things
- It only lasts a short time in the long run
- Life is amazing
- God knows what He's doing
- So excited about birth and meeting new baby
- Every step of the way is important, useful and necessary
- People really care and are doing the best they can with what they have
- Empathy
- Most belongings in life don't matter and it's important to let go
- Don't sweat the small stuff
- Success is measured in many different ways, most of which mean nothing
- Growing a baby isn't easy

- My body is amazing
- 2 grandmas passing makes new life that much greater
- Lots of people love me
- The world is very nice to you when you are pregnant
- I love chocolate
- How to feel nauseated but still eat

As I looked at this list, I realized the value of it for my learnings and future pregnancies. Writing out your learnings in any situation is helpful. It gives something to reference at any time.

In April, everything was ready to go: the birth pool and towels and everything needed for cutting the cord, as well as postpartum supplies—nipple cream, pump, swaddles, etc.

I had a dream on April 3rd that I had a baby while on the toilet and the baby just came right out and I called out to Jacob, "Hurry, I had a baby!" It was a girl in my dream.

I was having intense Braxton-Hicks contractions throughout the entire month of April. It was tiring. Sleeping was hit or miss. At night, I would wake up ready to go, fully energized at 4 in the morning. April 14th, I noted I was the only chiropractor on duty at the office that day, "Maybe baby will come out now."

On April 18th, I wrote, "Pretty hilarious when I was asked how far along I was at Wal-Mart. I told the lady my due date was April 5th to which she replied, 'Oh, you're getting close.' I said, 'It was 13 days ago.' She couldn't believe it. So funny to see the look on her face of complete awe and dumbstruck."

I realized I would miss my Grandma Grace's memorial service because the pregnancy kept going throughout the entire month of April. Her memorial was the end of April and I had tickets to go. I had fully expected I'd be going with a 3 week old baby. Being the baby was still in my belly, I wasn't allowed to fly.

April 19th: "God, give me the strength to make it through another day. Please help me to be more relaxed and trusting of Your will for me and new baby. Give me patience to make it through the night and to trust and have faith in your plans for us. Give me hope and joy and peace in my heart. I will exude joy and peace. I trust You, God and what You have in store for us. Amen."

I read some amazing articles and stories of women that just naturally go 43 and 44 weeks in their pregnancies and it's normal. Amish actually typically have babies at 43 weeks gestation. 10 Month Mamas was the name of one of the places I found support at the time. I read lots of inspiring stories of women who did not fall prey to induction. Research shows better outcomes with letting pregnancies go to "overdue" status and birthing spontaneously compared with induction. Again, this is my own personal experience. Every case is different and it's best to take an objective look at all of the factors involved. I suggest you read the article: "The Evidence on: Due Dates". This article was originally published in 2015 and last updated on November 24, 2019 by Rebecca Dekker, PhD, RN and Anna Bertone, MPH.

On April 30th, I noticed my first ever stretchmark and had another emotional moment. I had never had a stretchmark before. My high juice (out of a juicer) intake and cocoa butter had prevented that from ever occurring and here I am, 43 weeks and 4 days pregnant, discovering a stretchmark!

It was so important at this point to surround myself with supportive people. My father-in-law was very supportive and would make comments like, "You look great!" or "You are so lucky to be able to have babies so easily; there are so many people who can't get pregnant..." My grandpa was supportive as well. Annie was another big support. She kept encouraging me and telling me about how normal it was to carry longer than the standard 40 weeks. I found out from my mom and Jacob's mom, that both Jacob and I were carried a month past our due dates.

May 2nd: Mrs. Sharyn (a good friend) texted me that she'd been where I was twice. Six weeks overdue. That would mean 2 more weeks than me. It was helpful to hear I wasn't alone.

May 3rd: I noted I got my first gray hair… I then followed it by listing an entire page of things I was grateful for. Faith and surrender were on there.

11

RAE'S HOME BIRTH

"My baby will be born at the perfect time."

-ANONYMOUS

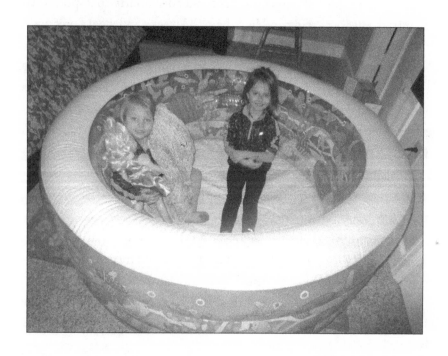

Written to Rae:

You were just born and I'm too excited to sleep. Everyone, including you is asleep right now. You were born 5/4/15 at 4:52 a.m. after 3 hours of labor. So, let's tell the story before the details get away from me:

1:40 a.m. May 4, 2015

"I'm definitely in labor," I said to myself as I struggle to stay comfortably sleeping. I decided to call Annie and I attempted to wake up Jacob 2 times but he was in such a deep sleep I was unsuccessful; that was probably for the best.

I went to the girls' bathroom as my bowels are completely evacuating themselves several times. I felt great relief every time.

Contractions are lasting a minute with 2 minutes in between.

I breathed deep breaths in through my nose, out through my mouth. It felt similar to deep menstrual-type sensations.

I got super excited because I saw the mucous plug had come out. When I checked myself, my cervix was very dilated (maybe 6-ish cm) and I could easily feel your head as well as the amniotic sac. I still had to stretch my finger in to get to it all. I figured there was a ways to go. But strangely enough, I did sense a bit of a pushing urge at the end of contractions.

Contractions were now 1 minute on, 1 minute off, and I decide it was time to wake Jacob up and he bolts into action immediately, setting everything up for the water birth.

I went to the kitchen and used the 2 counters kind of like parallel bars, straight-armed and just sagging into the contractions. Moving my hips forward feels best.

I put my phone on speaker and called Annie again around 2:30 a.m. and she answered. Jacob told her to come.

I felt like going to the girls' bathroom again to poop. I had the same urges to push through the end of contractions. I placed one hand on the bathtub and the other on the counter as I breathed through contractions.

At this point, Grace woke up and joined in. She wanted to be involved. She was so cute and excited that new baby was coming out soon.

She drew me a picture of our family with new baby. She also wrote me a note that says "I love Mom."

Annie arrived and spent some time getting the birth pool hotter as I was still laboring in the girls' bathroom.

I came out and drank water and labored between the kitchen counters. Annie put downward pressure on my shoulders and rubbed my spine. Felt great.

She asked me if I'd like to get in the pool at this point. I decided yes, if it was hot. And it was.

Felt fantastic to get in and I had what felt like a lengthy break in contractions. I began in an upright, seated position and switched to hands and knees as it felt better to be able to rock my hips. I felt like peeing so I got out and sat on the toilet. I had trouble initiating it so Annie turned water on to help. Then I had to poop again. Labored a bit on the toilet and had Jacob check me.

I wanted it to be done soon so I asked him how much longer. He said, "If your water breaks, it won't be long."

I cried and said, "My water doesn't break until the end of my births, remember?" I think this is the point I spoke about napping. I did hug pillows on the bed for a bit as I had my hips in the air rocking with contractions. There was definitely no napping.

I went to the dresser for 1 super uncomfortable contraction as I made my way to the bathroom. I had to pee and a bit more but pooping took place, not much though. As I sat on the toilet, I had 4 or 5 intense contractions and I knew I was having this baby soon. Annie suggested I get off the toilet and as I did, I had a really extended contraction that I had to put all of my focus into and actually ended up grabbing the sink and squatting up and down several times. Quite wildly. I said, "Baby's coming out!" I wanted to be in the pool but the contraction just wouldn't let up. Annie just guided me to the pool anyway and I immediately assumed an all fours position and began pushing you out.

"Counter pressure!" I told Jacob.

He said, "The amniotic sac ruptured, and you have just 3 more pushes." I felt every part of you moving down through my birth canal as your head emerged (a burning sensation) immediately followed by the shoulders, arms, torso and legs. I felt the rotation as you turned after your head was born. All of this was part of a single, continual contraction. I barely got a breath in as I pushed from the beginning to the end. You were born at 4:52 a.m.!

I was more relieved than I'd ever felt in my entire life. As you can see by the picture at the front of my book. That's Rae Rae, Grace standing by and Jacob with a bulb syringe for clearing the airway. He never had to use it.

You breathed right away and it sounded clear. You came out alert and eyes open, not crying or making any noise. Just content. You lay on my chest and were so relaxed.

Jacob clamped and cut the cord after 20 minutes when it stopped pulsating. My uterus felt "crampy" within minutes of your birth and I was able to push the placenta out maybe 25 minutes after you were born. Jacob assisted. Fastest placenta delivery I've had yet.

I got out of the birthing pool and took a shower. Felt strange not having you inside my belly. Haha. I loved it!

Daddy took you and put your diaper and first little newborn outfit on—a gray and white striped sleeper. He swaddled you. Grace put a little pink hat on your head.

I proceeded to feed you for the first time. You toyed with it a bit and then latched right on. You wanted to suck for a long stretch a bit later on. Maybe 15-20 minutes.

Barely a peep. You've been relaxed and content the whole day so far (it's 9 p.m. now as I continue writing).

Annie left at 6 a.m. after taking lots of pictures.

We were reminded of your initial attempt at entering the world March 7th when we looked at the date on the envelope I'd prepared for Annie when I had some false labor. You had not attempted to come again until today— the longest 2 months of my life.

Now I need to talk about this due date stuff. How stressful! Due date of April 5, 2015 (Easter Sunday) really messed with my mental state. Being pregnant wasn't the worst thing on me physically, but mentally/emotionally it was the hardest thing I've ever had to overcome. A 44-week long pregnancy. That's a long time. LMP (1st day of my last period) was June 29, 2014, making conception July 13, 2014, and the "due date" April 5, 2015. Never will I ever have a due date ever again. If I have any more babies, I will go with a "due season" that's a range of several weeks much, much, much, much later than the actual "due date."

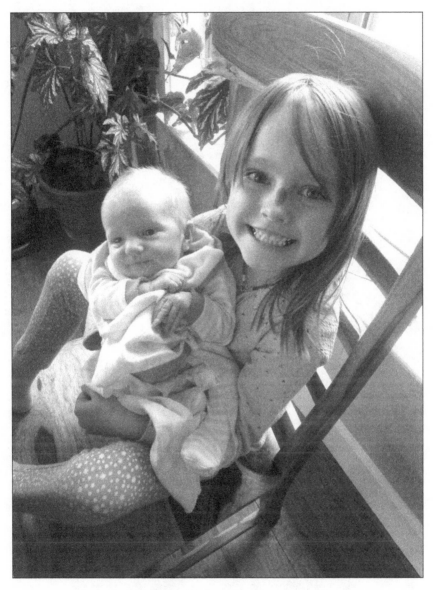

Grace holding Dakota Rae at 2 days old.

12

POSTPARTUM DEPRESSION

Overcoming feelings of inadequacy &
hopelessness

Dakota Rae was doing amazing. She was becoming "babywised" so I was actually getting some sleep for several hours at a time sometimes. I had mastitis from sleeping on my belly within the first couple weeks and it was a challenging time. It brought back memories of when I experienced mastitis with Grace. I remember having Grace bring Rae to me to feed her and then put her back in her crib. I felt alone much of this time. It completely knocked me out and I can't remember feeling that worn down and ill before. I had acupuncture that wiped out the mastitis completely.

I put a ton of pressure on myself to return to my pre-pregnant body within a short period of time. I immediately began a daily exercise routine. I did a post-pregnancy DVD that was an hour of ab, leg and arm strengthening. I did way too much, way too soon. I didn't give my body time to fully heal. Maybe because I felt pretty good after recovering from mastitis, I pushed myself to the max physically. I

DR. LAURA SIMS D.C.

started back at Curves (a gym for women) 5 days after her birth. This is definitely a pattern for me—to overdo it post-birth. You'd think I would have taken my own advice as it pertains to resting post-birth.

In addition to overdoing things physically, I also put pressure on myself to get back into the office. This was another pattern of mine that I work through and break in the years to come. By mid-June, I was already back in the office every afternoon and evening. The signs that it was too much, too soon, were showing up and I ignored them. I felt overwhelmed, but pushed though anyways. The pressure was building and I decided it would pass and I just kept up my typical high intensity, get it done attitude.

Then, my dog of 14 years, Madeline, was on death's doorstep. She'd been steadily declining for months and it was time to put her down. In June of 2015 she was put to rest. She'd been with me through everything: college, marriage, adopting another dog, Grace, Ada and now Rae. It was bittersweet in the end. I was so sad and glad all at the same time. She was no longer suffering. Ada said, "Mommy? Is Madeline playing with Grandma Grace in Heaven?"

I said "Yes!"

I'll never forget when my Grandma died on Christmas day, Ada said, "Grandma is playing with Jesus in Heaven."

This brought forward a great deal of grief and sadness. I attempted to move on. I thought I had. Eventually, with the daily exercise routine, work, all the recent deaths, and illness, it all finally caught up with me. I remember being on a road trip when Rae was six weeks old. We went from Colorado to Utah to Idaho to Montana to Wyoming and finally back home to Colorado. I was crying every day of the trip. Everything felt like the end of the world. I felt so much sadness. I was finally letting it all out. The full grieving that had never taken place with the deaths of Grandma and Madeline, the things I had felt around the last 2 months of my pregnancy with Rae... It was all coming out. We really had our minds made up that she was going to be early. Because of Grace being 11 days late and Ada being on her due date, the 3rd would be even sooner, right? There was so much unnecessary pressure and stress surrounding Rae's birth. Most of which was from myself. I did have lots of other things that I noted in my journal, like Jacob having trouble with the fact that I was still pregnant throughout the month of April and the pressures he felt being the only doctor in the office for most of April, May and half of June. The road trip was a great experience, but it just so happened to be when I had a total melt down.

This is the time I would have counseled myself to seek help. With what I know now, and all my therapy experience—both education-wise and personally seeking therapy years later—that would have been a great first step. The reason this would have helped, is because it would have been an opportunity for me to work through all of the feelings I was experiencing. I can remember thinking that therapy was for other people, not me. There was also a lot of stress stemming from a non-profit organization I'd began in 2014 that I needed to do a 990 for. I learned how to do it all on my own (99 page instruction manual) and went through all the bank statements and categorized everything appropriately. It was a lot of pressure. I was picturing the worst if things weren't done correctly. It was nuts. This began before Rae's birth, and it may very well have had a lot to do with why I was pregnant so long. I tell all the details of my experience here in hopes it will help you in the event that you feel a similar sort of overwhelm.

Feelings of failure, "not good enough" and sadness coursed through me. It was too much. I didn't reach out for support from anyone other than Jacob. He was also at the end of his rope. Everything exploded on me at once, and I felt completely alone, like I was the only person who'd ever felt this way in the history of the world. I thought with everything I'd accomplished and where I was in life, I should have felt great. So, yes, therapy would have been helpful here because I so desperately needed to hear another person tell me that I would make it through this. A therapist that accepted me as I was, however broken, and help me navigate through the hopelessness. And help me to get grounded. Another human being that could have been a sounding board for me. I had a sense that I needed to slow down and allow myself to process through these difficult emotions. It would have helped me to understand my needs on a deeper level and helped me to take action.

This is also where self-care comes into the equation. Doing things nutritionally to fuel myself in a loving way. Taking more baths. Sitting out in the sun. Getting more rest. Having the occasional pedicure. Taking the girls on long walks/runs with Grace biking beside me and the other girls in the jogger. I started slowly incorporating things that fed my soul. It was incredibly fulfilling to me. Spiritual replenishment was helpful as well through prayer and intentionality. The thing that made the biggest impact for me is in the following chapter.

If I could tell my 32-year-old self anything, it would be that you didn't do anything wrong. I love you. You're magnificent and you are beautiful. You can release the judgements.

13

SIMPLIFY

*"Minimalism is the intentional promotion
of the things we most value and the removal
of anything that distracts us from it."*

- JOSHUA BECKER

*"Simplicity involves unburdening your life,
and living more lightly with fewer distractions
that interfere with a high quality life, as
defined uniquely by each individual."*

- LINDA BREEN PIERCE 1947

This is such an exciting topic for me! It played an important role surrounding pregnancy, motherhood and life in general. The journey of simplifying my life began during Rae's pregnancy. I was becoming overwhelmed with my schedule, my duties, cleaning all the time and not having any time for the things that were really important to me: Family, Fun, Travel & Freedom!

It all began with an enormous closet declutter. I went into my closet and could barely move around, it was so jam-packed. I didn't have a large closet to begin with and I had really stuffed it to the gills! I had clothing I'd worn in high school and college still in there, sentimental items, bedding, shoes, books, and much more.

I decided that if I hadn't used an item in the last year, it was leaving my life! I ended up with 6 large black garbage bags to donate, all just from my closet. It was hard to believe that much could fit within my 3' X 4' closet. That catapulted me into major decluttering. I went to my bathroom and came out with 2 boxes full of products and hair accessories and towels we hadn't used in over a year. I went into the attic and decluttered all my unpacked boxes from our move 3 years prior. This was intense. There were lots of photos that I ended up digitizing and displaying my favorite ones. I dug through tons of books, stuff from my childhood and sports equipment. That was a dirty job! I even went into my collection of textbooks and notes from chiropractic school that I hadn't cracked open since I was a student. I attacked my nightstand. All that remained was my lamp, my phone charger and my journal. I emptied my half of the dresser. I no longer needed the extra space now that I'd removed 80% of the excess items from my closet. I easily fit all my shoes, my capsule wardrobe and my jewelry in my closet, as well as my yoga mat and travel bag. A single purse remained. I literally and mentally felt lighter. It was a huge boost to my honing in on what was truly important in my life.

I then went to the kitchen. I found so many items we hadn't used in the past year. Half our pantry was either expired or stuff we hadn't touched in over a year. By this point, I'd decluttered and deep-cleaned my bedroom, bathroom and the kitchen. I was feeling on top of the world. That physical clutter was sucking my energy and I hadn't even realized it until it was gone. Removing the things that did not bring value to my life transformed my entire being. I can remember taking car load after car load to our local charity shop. The first run through the entire house resulted in 6 full car loads.

The living room was easy. The junk drawer and electronics cabinet took some time. It's amazing how many unnecessary cords and accessories we hold on to "just in case." It really made me re-evaluate my purchases. I cleared out the laundry room, the mudroom, the linen closet, my desk, the coat closet, the garage and the outside of our home.

Lastly, I made my way through the girls' rooms. Rae's room was the easiest because she was an infant that didn't care about stuff. So, I excised the 20 extra blankets she didn't need, and the extra clothes I'd saved from Grace and Ada that Rae wouldn't need because she'd been gifted so many new clothes. I removed extra toys. In fact, she had no toys, except a few stuffed animals. I had simplified her room the most and it was the room everyone wanted to hang out in. It had a comfy couch, a nice rug, the diaper changing area with clothes storage and her crib. That's it!

Her closet had become my office shelving area that contained all the records from 2008 - present. I digitized all of it except the 3 most recent tax returns, important documents such as birth certificates and passports, 3 years of receipts, employee time cards (2 years) and certificates from college. It took me several days to digitize all of that, but with a high efficiency scanner, it was totally doable. With a completely clear closet, I stuck the wardrobe furniture piece inside to be able to be Rae's future toy storage area. I sold the spare 2 chiropractic tables we'd had in her closet and made some good money!

On to Grace and Ada's room. Grace is what we refer to as the "bag lady." She loves collecting stuff and never gets rid of anything, including trash. I approached carefully. I decided it was time for a wakeup call and I had her and Ada grab all of their things and put them all in a pile on the floor of their bedroom. There was no walking space once they had everything out! This was really helpful for her to see how much stuff she had. The girls got to work, and with lots of help from me, whittled their belongings down by half. It cleared up so much space that the girls both noted how much more area they had to play.

I highly recommend not touching kids' things until you've decluttered all of your belongings first. Set the example. Then assist them. Jacob was the most challenging and after years of setting the example, I'm happy to say that he's decluttered many of his belongings that don't bring value to his life, with no involvement from me.

This is an on-going process. It took a few months to get through everything. Then, I did another declutter sweep and another and another, until I felt like I got to that sweet spot where all of my surroundings brought value or were useful to us and I felt like I was living my best life ever!

The physical simplification is easy compared with decluttering your mental, emotional and spiritual life. The mental aspect takes time and awareness of inner self-talk—the things you communicate in regards to yourself, the judgements. My therapist took me through an exercise where I carried a heavy rock for a while. It continued to get heavier and was a burden. She told me I could release the judge at any point I felt ready. Let go of the JUDGE! I chucked it with all my strength. I felt so much lighter. Finding that inner peace. Listening to that inner knowing. Coming to a place where you are your authentic self and nothing going on in the external can even touch you. You're in total love, peace, compassion, joy and acceptance of yourself and others. This is difficult for me with my ego trying to intervene with everything. When I'm in a space of full acceptance, I'm loving every part of myself no matter what. I'm aware of the inherent power within and following my life purpose. I am taking action steps inside and out to support my dreams. What my spiritual growth looks like is me letting go and surrendering the judgements and things that prevent me from reaching my souls purpose. Giving it over to God. Letting go and then letting go some more. It's a never-ending process for me, clearing out the mental clutter and physical clutter. Once I decluttered my life and my schedule, I had space for what matters most to me.

In *The 5 Regrets of the Dying*, written by hospice nurse Bronnie Ware, she says the 5 regrets are:

1. I wish I'd had the courage to live a life true to myself, not the life others expected of me.
2. I wish I hadn't worked so hard.
3. I wish I'd had the courage to express my feelings.
4. I wish I'd stayed in touch with my friends.
5. I wish that I had let myself be happier.

All of these things are choices, choices that I've decided to act upon immediately! Relationships are so vital. And living a life true to yourself! That's where my list of things that follow my beliefs comes into play. We've communicated our beliefs within our business and how we feel about the innate power of the body to heal itself without drugs and surgery. We've been able to include the girls in our practice and work. Giving ourselves all day Friday, Saturday and Sunday to be with the family. Monday mornings as well. I'm choosing happiness more and more with every passing day. This didn't all happen overnight. There were many days in the initial years that we worked crazy hours. We were on the same mission. Many things have come to be because we've worked together as a team. What began as hundreds of thousands of dollars in debt has ended with living a debt-free, mortgage-free lifestyle. It's created a lot of freedom and it wasn't easy. All good things require hard work.

Did I mention that we decided to build a tiny home? My dream was to live simply in a tiny home one day. Here's our 26-foot tiny home. It has everything a normal home has. This includes a kitchen, living room, a washing machine, two loft bedrooms, a bathroom and a twin bedroom on the main level. Lots of blood (Jacob put a nail through the web of his hand), sweat and tears. It was worth it. It is now completely outfitted with solar. A Tipi sits adjacent to the tiny home on its own platform. You can do anything. Coming into agreement and working together toward a common goal is what produced this result. It's really the same concept with the businesses and our girls. Experiences are special and we make the most out of this limited time we have with the girls in their childhood.

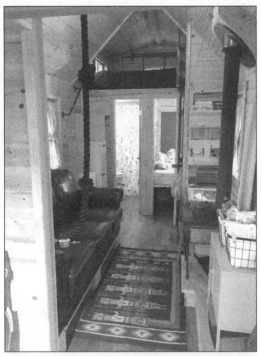

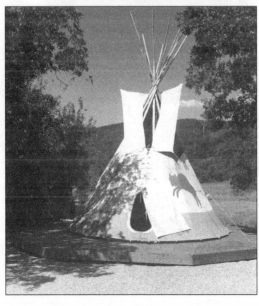

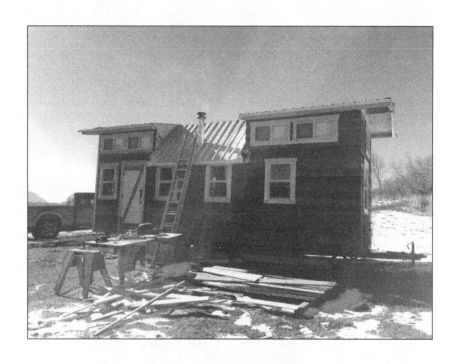

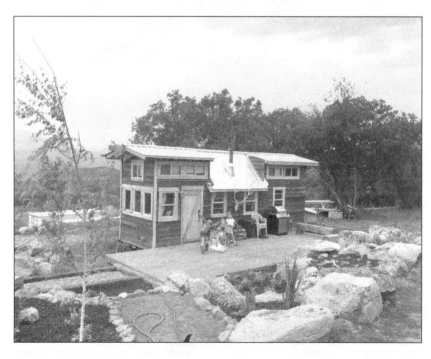

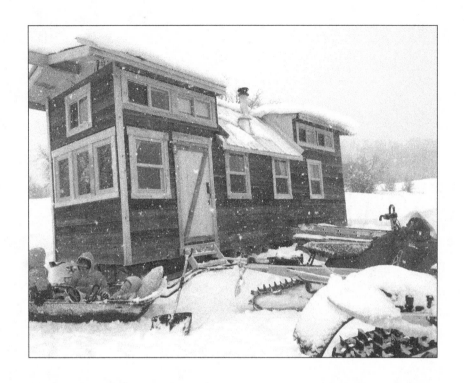

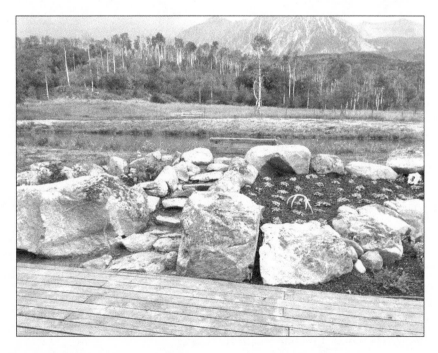

14

UNEXPECTED MISCARRIAGE

"The authentic self is the soul made visible."

-SARAH BAN BREATHNACH

This is a difficult chapter to write. After a life-altering experience, I can say I feel stronger, more in tune with the blessings in my life and in a state of acceptance.

It all began with the onset of my Soul-Centered Living year 2 program when they announced we would be working on a project that was a sacred yes for me. A sacred yes is something that calls out to you. It's a deep inner knowing. When it comes to light, it's an opportunity to get out of your comfort zone. It's apart of your purpose for being. I had a deep desire to write my story. When I say "my story," I really mean everything I've experienced with pregnancy, birth & motherhood. I immediately started in on it and upon reading my journals from Grace's, Ada's and Rae's pregnancies and births, I realized I wasn't finished having babies. I'd never closed the door on the idea, and writing this ignited my soul. I realized having another baby was and is a sacred yes for me.

My inner dialogue up to this point had been, "You can't have another because of the businesses," or, "You have too much responsibility as it is," and, "I'm so content with the 3 girls; why mess with that?" I was reminded of the book *The 5 Regrets of the Dying* by Bronnie Ware. She was a hospice nurse for 30 years and put all of her learnings into this book. The main regret was: "I wish I hadn't worked so hard." Upon reflection of that concept, I was convinced that having another baby was the best idea ever!

Looking through all of our photos from just Jacob and I and the dogs to having 1, 2 and then 3 babies to the present moment with our beautiful family, all I felt was immense gratitude. Our life has been and is amazingly vibrant and beautiful. We were so blessed to be where we were and to have the family and friends and so many factors aligning so perfectly. We had just renewed our vows in May 2018 in front of 45 of our closest family and friends. Our family had overcome adversity and attack within our business and marriage had been put through the biggest challenge to date. Throughout 2017, we had experienced blackmail within the business and me not knowing what was going on because I did not have a physical presence in our 2nd office at that time. It was confusing and ultimately led to couples counseling and after a year and a half, a renewing of our commitment to one another. Our marriage and our family were worth it and nothing was going to break us apart. I feel this is necessary in being able to grasp the struggle and reaching bottom before coming into the light again. We were changed. For the better. Our love for one another had never been stronger.

When I approached my husband about baby #4, he was ALL IN! I'd been tracking my cycle and knew exactly when I was going to ovulate in November 2018. It was the day before Thanksgiving! So, we planned to have a romantic moment that morning. So, coming back to that experiment I spoke of in a previous chapter about how to up the chances of having a boy. We decided we were going to try it. I also read that if you do it doggy style on the day of ovulation that supposedly increases the chances of having a boy. I laughed when I first heard this. Then I looked up all the statistics and it's actually proven by Dr. Shettles in 1970. We were happy to have either, but thought it wouldn't hurt to give the method a try. The lead up seemed to take forever. Finally the day arrived and we went for it!

It was only a matter of 2-3 days and I felt very pregnant. I actually felt implantation. I've read about women being able to feel this and had never experienced it for myself. I thought they were just imagining things. Now that I've felt it myself, I realize how real it is. I felt extremely warm and fuzzy and like my body was beginning to create something amazing!

I knew I was pregnant and wanted a pregnancy test to validate it! I purchased several. The early response tests that say "know 6 days before missed period!" all came out negative. I wasted so much money on tests that kept saying I wasn't pregnant. I decided to grab a 25 pack from Amazon for $7.99 after wasting $40-50 dollars on all the tests I had taken up until the point of my missed period. The day my period was supposed to start came and went and I just wanted a positive test already! I had just returned from a trip and took one that night. Negative...

I woke up the next morning and told my husband that your pee is the strongest in the morning so this test would surely be positive! I peed on that darn stick for what felt like the 100th time and waited the suggested 3 minutes. Negative.

I started to cry and literally broke down about the fact that I knew deep inside I was pregnant and why were these tests all negative? It was somewhat comical. I began getting ready for the day and glanced at the test after getting out of the shower. There was a line! An extremely faint pink line. I thought I might have been making it up at first and stared at it for the longest time. I changed the angle at which I was looking at it and positioned it every which way. There was a definite line. I yelled for Jacob to come. He saw it too! We were pregnant!

We had a mini celebration in the bathroom and talked about when this baby would come. Would it decide to be a 10-month baby or on-time? Either way, we'd made up our minds to tell people a season for the due date. "The baby is coming in the autumn," or "the baby will definitely be here by 2020," which was over a year away.

We planned a party for December 22nd to surprise our friends and family with the news. We didn't even tell the girls. My grandpa bought a flight from Canada—12 hours of travel. My parents, sister and 1 of my brothers were coming! Jacob's family would be there! I purchased 40 Christmas cards that announced "Baby #4" and "Gender reveal coming soon!" I strategically mailed them so no one would receive a card prior to the party.

I think I'm the most impatient person I know. It was the biggest secret I'd ever had to keep and the days seemed to drag on forever. I just wanted to blurt it out to the world! We were so happy and looking forward to this addition to our family! The joys of pregnancy. I was glowing, and tired all the time, and sleeping 10-12 hours at night. It was fabulous. I was craving protein and couldn't get enough of these vegan maple sausages!

Ovia Pregnancy app became my daily go-to. I started using it at 3 weeks and 6 days pregnant. I recorded how I was feeling every morning. Common things for me were: fatigue, tender breasts, increased appetite, increased thirst, increased urination, etc. I also tracked my moods: happy, supported, sad, weepy, loving, joyful, peaceful, calm, anxious, depressed, etc. I tracked my sleep patterns as well as my prenatal vitamin. I'd been taking a prenatal 3 months prior to getting pregnant and every day of my pregnancy. Every bit of this pregnancy felt similar, if not identical, to the first 3. I continued to be active. I ran 3 miles a few times. Prior to becoming pregnant, I had been training for a marathon and commonly ran 10-15 miles at a time. During this pregnancy I mostly walked and started in on some yoga. It all felt so good. I got adjusted almost every day and had Swedish massages every other week.

Part of my 2nd year project for my Master's program was running a marathon. I easily transitioned that into the marathon of pregnancy! It became all about radiant health and fully embracing my pregnant self. This involved upping my self-care, nutrition and activities. I wrote out an ideal scene for radiant health as well as a living vision I will include in the back of this book. Everything was on track and I was more accepting and trusting of my body and my whole being than ever before.

I bought the belly belt to extend the amount of time I could wear my pants. I got a few maternity clothes in preparation. I also bought the cutest baby Christmas socks. I ordered a blank puzzle for the party. The girls and I drew with permanent markers a beautiful heart with the message "Surprise! We are pregnant with baby #4!" I wrote in the message after we did the heart so the girls wouldn't see that until the party.

Ovia kept me updated on what was forming and developing every week. By the time of the party, baby was the size of a blueberry and baby's heart had formed. It had a nervous system and a face. Arm and leg buds were forming.

Party time! It was finally here. I'd felt some anxiety leading up to the party. People were changing their plans here and there and ultimately we ended up with a decent sized group. My grandpa flew into our little mountain town the day before and we made sure he was comfortable in the guest bed with plenty of oxygen and chocolates. My parents arrived the day of the party. Jacob's parents and sister and the girls' cousin were there as well. Finally! We can do the puzzle. We corralled everyone into the living room and hand out 4 envelopes containing a quadrant of the puzzle. They started building. Ten minutes went by and I wondered if we needed to get an easier puzzle. Sixty-three pieces was taking forever for them to build. I began filming it with my phone which I placed on my desk so there was a view of the entire living room.

The puzzle was completed and Jacob's mom read the message, "Surprise! We are pregnant with baby #4!" Pause… They all registered that I was pregnant and the hugs and joyful yelling began! My mom was surprised. Jacob's dad started crying. My mother-in-law wanted to know the due date. To which I said, "Autumn."

My mom and she were not accepting of this reply. They asked, "No, really, when is the baby due?"

Jacob told them before 2020. My grandpa made the sweetest toast known to mankind, saying he was so excited for his 4th great-granddaughter! We all, except me and the kids, had champagne. It was a beautiful, joyful moment and a holiday feast followed.

We discussed SneakPeek, an at-home finger prick, gender test. It gets mailed in at week 9 and they test your blood for male DNA. If present, it's a boy. If not, it's a girl. We'd never found out the gender before and this was actually something I had discussed with Jacob prior to getting pregnant. I told him I wanted to find out this time so we could mentally prepare. We would do this test on January 11, 2019 and have the results emailed to us within a matter of days.

We celebrated over the next several days. Everyone went home after the Christmas holiday.

I talked with the girls about new baby and they were so excited. Ada had been asking for a baby. Grace had wanted a baby for a while. Rae Rae wanted a "girl baby." We were on a high.

December 26, 2018 I began feeling intense pain in my left kidney and I was having body aches. On top of that, my throat burned and was so sore that I could not speak. I was bed-ridden for days. I wondered why I wasn't feeling better. It continued to get worse and I felt sicker than I'd ever been in my life. Jacob was waiting on me and bringing tea, as well as natural remedies and soup.

I marked in my pregnancy app that I was experiencing pelvic pain and cramping and spotting. I felt worse and worse. I couldn't sleep at night. I had intense pain all over, and I couldn't eat.

December 30th rolled around and I finally get out of bed because I needed to go to the bathroom. It was the evening. A large amount of blood fell out of me. I knew this was *not* normal. I showed Jacob and he said, "You're going to be okay." Then, only 30 minutes later, it felt like I was in labor. I got in the shower because there was so much blood. I was doubled over and sobbing at this point. I knew the pregnancy was ending early. Really early—7 weeks and 2 days. I sat on the toilet and the sac fell out of me. I picked it up and held the baby. I could see the head, body and arm/leg buds. The sac was the size of my palm and the baby was 1/4 of that. I felt a rush of peaceful sensations traverse through my body from top to bottom. It was the sensation of pregnancy leaving me. I felt lightheaded. I had lost a lot of blood; it was basically pouring out of me. I immediately lay down, bawling my eyes out. The thoughts running through my brain included things like: "Why?" "What did I do to cause this?" "How did I not see this coming?" "What went wrong?" Plus extreme sadness for the loss of baby #4.

My husband and I talked about it. He assured me there was something not right with the baby and my body was smart and knew it needed to end the pregnancy. The baby couldn't sustain life. He said that this was the best thing that could happen in the event that the baby could not sustain life. He was holding me for hours. We got close that night. I felt more connected to him than I ever had. He cried and he rarely shows emotion. I could see the sadness in his eyes. We were both devastated and in a state of disbelief. I was starving after not eating all day. Jacob made me the best soup I've ever tasted—vegetable broth and onions. Just what I needed.

He said a prayer for the baby's spirit. We cried some more. I actually felt quite clear at this point. I really opened up about everything I was feeling and experiencing. I went into my intentions moving forward. I went through a range of emotions from denial to anger to hurt to love. That night, I thought to myself, the "why" doesn't matter. It doesn't change what happened. The baby had still left my body, and I came to a place of acceptance.

The following morning, I woke up crying. Before my eyes opened, I was crying, grieving the loss of this beautiful soul. I announced to my family what had happened. My mom and sister took immediate action and started driving out to support me. It was an extremely snowy day and it took them the entire day to get to me. I still had huge blood clots coming out, the size of gumballs, multiple times throughout the day.

Grace asked me if the baby was in Heaven. I said, "Definitely." She cried. I cried.

Rae Rae questioned it. She said, "The baby isn't in your belly?" I told her no. She went on about her day. At 3 years old, it's a tough concept to grasp.

Ada didn't talk. I asked her what she was feeling. She asked several questions like, "Where is the baby?" and "Why did the baby leave your belly?"

My spiritual mentor called me after I texted her about what had happened. She was so helpful, listening to me, talking to me about how the baby had served a purpose. Albeit short, the baby had come to do what it needed to do. We talked about acceptance and sadness. She brought up several quotes that were helpful. I was so glad to be able to have that right away, especially after announcing to the world that I was pregnant and this happening 8 days later. I felt like I'd disappointed everyone. I forgave myself for that and all the judgement swirling around in my brain. Things like, "I stayed in the hot tub too long," or "I wasn't active enough," or "I was too stressed out," or "I drank too much chai tea." The quicker you can bust through those untruths, the better. It does not help to beat yourself up about something that is caused by chromosomal abnormalities 75% of the time and chronic disease 15% of the time, leaving 10% for things like alcohol and drugs. It's *not* your fault! I realized I could not have judgement and freedom at the same time.

My mom and sister finally arrived and I was super sick and feverish. It had been 24 hours since the miscarriage and I was very unwell. I could finally speak again but my body was not doing well. They sprang into action and got me essential oils in the diffuser and Quick Response (a garlic, echinacea blend) tea, and soup. My mom adjusted me. (It's handy having chiropractors for parents). My sister and mom hugged me. I saw the positive pregnancy tests sitting on my bedside table and totally lost it. The feminine energy was helpful, the total support regardless of my state.

I decided to burn the puzzle and remove anything that reminded me of the baby I had just lost. The maternity stuff I'd just bought went into the bottom drawer of my closet, put away for a future pregnancy. "We'll have another," I thought.

That night after the loss, I was so ill that I gladly took some ibuprofen. I woke up around 3 a.m. when I needed to pee. I went to the bathroom and almost passed out. The heavy blood loss was catching up to me. I lay on the bathroom floor trying to regain my composure. I was hallucinating and everything was spinning and closing in around me. After a few minutes, I got up and ran to the bed. I didn't want to not make it to my bed. I was in the throes of sadness and illness. It was miserable. My kidney pain had gone away, but I was feeling my throat and chest as well as body aches. My uterus was cramping big time. I can only describe it as being 100 times worse than a period. It was a different thing altogether. There's really no comparison.

I started researching on the internet where I learned you bleed for 14 days and the recovery from a miscarriage can take weeks, if not months, to fully heal. I also read some encouraging things. It's easier to get pregnant and not miscarry after a miscarriage. Some women get pregnant a couple weeks after a miscarriage. You get your period 4-6 weeks post miscarriage. I was hopeful.

I watched several YouTube videos on miscarriage and listened to all these women talk about their experiences with it. That really helped. I felt like all these women came out of the woodwork about their miscarriages when I opened up about mine—family members, friends, people I barely knew, even our nanny. She told me she got pregnant with her 3rd 2 months after miscarrying. It was so encouraging to know I'm not alone. It's actually surprising, the statistics on miscarriage. On the Mayo Clinic website, it sites: "10 to 20% of known pregnancies end in miscarriage. But the actual number is likely higher because many miscarriages occur so early in pregnancy that a woman doesn't realize she's pregnant. Miscarriage is a somewhat loaded term — possibly suggesting that something was amiss in the carrying of the pregnancy. This is rarely true. Most miscarriages occur because the fetus isn't developing normally."

I was on a mission to heal! I didn't go into the offices at all that entire week. My mom and sister were bringing me all kinds of healing remedies and teas and nutrient-rich foods. Protein is important after a miscarriage. As a vegan, the protein-rich sources that were easiest were: vegan protein shakes, bars, lentils, beans, tofu and protein-rich soups. I really wanted broth.

Another thing I experienced, along with the intense pain in my lower abdomen, was an enlarged uterus. My belly had not looked pregnant before, but now it did. For 10 days I had a little bump. My abdomen was really swollen as my uterus was contracting back down to size and my body was naturally expelling everything that had to do with pregnancy—lots and lots of bleeding, way more than after a natural childbirth. It was like having multiple periods in a row and at the same time. Very intense. I feel like this part of miscarriage was a bit sugarcoated in my online reading. It's really challenging. Right when you think the bleeding is almost over with, you get an outpouring of clots and more blood. I went through two large packages of pads. It's really best to use pads so you avoid infection, and NO sex for two weeks. For real. You won't feel like having sex anyway. Your man will need to be understanding of this. Any intercourse is going to lead to possible infection. It's not worth it. This is a time to focus on you and your healing.

I really felt like being by myself after the initial few days of support. I needed time to process. Thankfully, I had one of my University of Santa Monica weekends a week after the miscarriage. I fully processed and opened up about what happened. I felt heard and understood and like I was in the exact right place that weekend. I was able to see the opportunity in what had happened with the baby. The opportunity to help other women and write about my experience.

I felt so strong two weeks after the miscarriage and ready for what was to come. I was finally feeling back to normal physically. It honestly felt like I was going to be recovering for forever. It had been super intense up until the previous couple days. Now it was about a fresh start. It was a new year. It was possible I would get my period in a couple weeks and be pregnant on the next ovulation day a couple weeks later.

Love Letter to Baby:

> January 9, 2019
> Dear Baby,
>
> I love you from the depths of my soul. We (you and me) were one for 7 weeks and 2 days. Thank you God for allowing me the opportunity! Baby, you are very dear to me and I love you. We were so overjoyed when I found out you were growing inside of me. The girls love you too. Grace asked me if you were in Heaven. I told her, "Definitely!" The experience of losing you was challenging and I am in acceptance of it all and the purpose you served to bring our family closer. Your father and I are more connected and he is sad by your not being with us anymore. I know your spirit is still with us. I treasure you. I am excited for the day I meet you in Heaven. For now, you have fun with Hunter, Madeline and Great-Grandma Grace! I will love you forever.
>
> Love,
> Your Mom

15

HOPE

"I dwell in possibility."

-EMILY DICKINSON

Two and a half months later, following my 2nd period since the miscarriage, I was pregnant! This was the happiest news we'd had for a long time. We were hesitant to shout it from the rooftops until I was further along. I was feeling extreme nausea. It reminded me of when I was pregnant with Ada and had a tiny window of feeling nauseated and vomiting. The difference now was that the nausea lasts for 15+ weeks. It was as if it was never going to end. I didn't throw up, but I was starving and nauseated all at the same time. It was like torture. My belly and entire body were expanding as per my usual growth during pregnancy. Nothing helped with this wretched feeling. It got so bad that I couldn't even drink plain water any more. I tried Preggie Pop Drops, root beer, sparkling water, crackers, lots of ginger chews, bland foods, sea bands, acupuncture, eating smaller meals more frequently, calm-a-tum tincture for morning sickness and apple cider vinegar. You name it, I tried it. Sea bands were the only thing that took the edge off.

I made it to the 9 week mark. I'd saved the SneakPeek test that I had never gotten to use. I pricked my finger and put about 12 drops of blood into this tiny plastic vile. I mailed it into SneakPeek, eagerly awaiting the news of girl or boy. A couple days later, the result was in my inbox. I was hesitant and nervous to open it. Later, when I was on the phone with Jacob, I opened it and found out the baby was a GIRL! I was relieved. Maybe because I felt like I had that gender down. I did feel a little twinge of, "I hope this isn't a disappointment to him." Jacob was elated. We eagerly anticipated the arrival of a baby girl. As for our experimentation with timing of conception and positions, it didn't work for us and that was just fine.

This was the first time we'd found out the gender before the birth. I decided to make it really fun for the girls and we had a black, gender reveal balloon. Grace popped it and pink confetti goes everywhere. Grace and Ada had a moment of, "I thought it would be a boy!" and Rae didn't understand at first but got really excited when she realized she was getting a baby sister just like she wanted. I texted the video of this to all our friends and family.

I woke up the next morning wondering about the validity of the gender reveal test. I googled it and found some reviewers noted that it was wrong for them. I ordered 2 more tests and took them. Same results. It was definitely a girl! This was so cool. Four girls. The symptoms continued and I came to a point where I really began to embrace my pregnancy, regardless of what I was experiencing physically. This is where my ideal scene and living vision (in the back of this book) helped.

At 11 weeks along, I begin to think about what I'll need to get for her. I gave away most of the girls baby stuff. I started to shop online. I put everything I would need for her in my Amazon cart. We spent many hours going over names. I had a baby bump and my clothing became uncomfortable. I started wearing maternity clothes by this time. Week 11, I felt her moving inside of me, like fluttering. I wrote in my journal that her daddy was spending time talking to her and rubbing over my belly and playing with her. I still had zero relief from the intense nausea. I started to wonder if everything was okay.

Week 14, I went to see a midwife. This was my first experience with a midwife. She did the Doppler ultrasound and the girls and I got a black and white video of the baby on the TV screen. She wiggled and moved all around. Her tiny arms and legs were so cutely punching and kicking. Her heartbeat was so strong and loud. It was 152 beats per minute. The midwife said, "You've got a perfectly healthy baby in there," and "Sounds like a very nice baby!" I was relieved and I texted Jacob the video of her heartbeat. I had lab work done and everything came back normal. Better than normal! Even the chromosomal testing ruled out any abnormalities. The blood work the lab did also confirmed a female gender. Waiting for the results was nerve-wracking, nevertheless, I was moving right along.

The girls were fighting over whose room the baby would sleep in. They all wanted her crib in their room. I hadn't ordered everything yet, but it was all in the ready. All I needed to do was click "buy." I was searching for a doula nearby, and could not locate a single one. I reached out to Annie even though she lived over an hour away from our home. She was all in! I told her I would definitely call her at the first signs of labor so she would make it in time. We knew my births were becoming faster and faster.

I was just about halfway into the pregnancy when we all went to Montana for a family vacation. When we got back from our trip, I found out that my school required that I see a doctor because there is going to be some "release" work during my last class. I'm about to go through my final week long practicum for year 2 of my University of Santa Monica program. I'm not allowed to know the details of what we will be doing, all I know is I need a doctors note. So, I decided to see the doctor that worked in the same building as the midwife I had recently seen. I hadn't planned to see her or any other health care provider ever again. We had intended to do the same thing we'd always done with having a home birth, with only our family and our doula. I call my school and tell them I've never been to a doctor before and described my situation. They insisted, so I set up the appointment.

Week 17 and 4 days into my pregnancy, I meet the obstetrician that will be evaluating me and explain my situation. She asks me how the pregnancy has been going and I explain to her everything I've been experiencing. She then takes me into the room with the doppler ultrasound and puts the gel on my lower abdomen. The ultrasound was underway. I fully anticipated seeing the baby flipping around in there and hearing a solid heartbeat. Silence... I immediately asked why I didn't see her moving on the screen and why I couldn't hear her heart beating. She told me it might be the machine.

We went to the other room. The 2nd ultrasound machine had the same result. I saw her lifeless body inside me. The heart I once saw expanding and contracting was completely still. Measurements of her skull and leg bone are taken to determine her age. She comes in as a week and a half younger (16 weeks gestational age) then where I am in my pregnancy. My heart is racing. I try to recall what I was doing a week and a half ago.

A week and a half ago we were in Montana. It all comes flooding back. It was the day our raft capsized and we almost died in the Madison River. It hits me. This intense wave of, "This can't be happening!?" It doesn't feel real. The kids are quickly ushered to the waiting room. I began sobbing. "Why?! I was so far along. She was healthy. Why God, Why?!"

I begin to ask the Doctor questions. I asked her if this was a result of the accident? She looked at all of the data before her; my history, the measurements from my first ultrasound a few weeks prior and the measurements from today, gestational age and how far along I am in this pregnancy. She responded. "There's a direct correlation with the date of the accident and the date her heart stopped. We know her heart stopped beating a week and a half ago according to her measurements." I asked how often they see this happen. She shook her head. "This happens about one time per year. It's very uncommon, especially with how far along you are. There's a 1% chance this will happen at this stage of pregnancy." I was not sure how I felt about this. All I know is that no matter what anyone is saying to me right now, it doesn't help. I wanted to reverse what had happened. Go back to that day on the raft and not get on it in the first place. I wanted her to be alive right now.

I journaled about that day in Montana where we rented a raft and set out as a family on the Madison River. This is a family-friendly river. It was a clear, sunny day and the river was a relaxing experience. We were fishing and enjoying our time together.

Several hours into our rafting experience, our raft got caught in a strainer and violently flipped. The girls, Jacob, and our friend TJ and I were at the mercy of this wickedly strong undercurrent churning us all about. My only thought at this time was to grab Ada and Rae, who had been in the back of the raft with me pre-flip. I propelled myself down river and as I came up out of the water, there they both were. I grabbed Ada's life vest with my right hand and Rae's with my left and I started swimming like the dickens to get us to shore. It seemed impossible as the river took us wherever it wanted. TJ came to us and grabbed Rae. I told Ada to grab my neck and I started swimming with everything I had. I felt like I couldn't breathe. The water was frigid, between 30 and 40 degrees. For the first time, I thought about her—the baby in my belly. I thought, "Is she okay in there?" I saw the overturned raft and swam as hard as I could to get to it. I finally made it and grabbed the side handle. Jacob popped out from underneath. I asked him what I should do. He was in shock. He'd been underneath the raft this whole time. It felt like it had been several minutes since we had all been tossed in the river.

None of us were able to touch the bottom of the very deep river. There had been a lot of melt off and the rivers were high. Ada started shouting that we could get to the shore. I let go of the raft, and again, swam with everything I had. My feet finally touched the ground and I propelled Ada toward shore and watched as she got up on the bank. My feet were battered and bruised as I scrambled up and out of the water. I'd been kicking hard in the water and I must have injured them throughout the entire incident.

I was on shore now and looked down river. I saw Grace had made it to the bank, but she was quite a ways down river. I looked across the river and saw TJ holding Rae Rae.

The night following the capsizing, I didn't sleep at all. I was replaying it in my mind. It had all happened so fast, and we were powerless to stop it. I had such a clear picture in my mind of Rae's face before the accident. She was smiling so cutely. I had reached for her as I realized what was about to happen. That's when the raft had rolled, dumping all of us into the frigid waters that sucked us under. I had never experienced that feeling of utter powerlessness. The raft had flipped and my girls' lives were in danger. Including the life of our unborn child. As I lay in bed, I realized how beat up my body felt. The next morning, I could barely walk. My feet and lower legs were cut up and bruised so badly that each step was excruciating. I spent the entire next day in bed. We were all shaken up.

My mind never went there, never to the place of the possibility of something being wrong with the baby. A couple of days later, I thought I felt her move. I was recovering. I noticed that my appetite was lower. When I looked in the mirror I noticed I was not much bigger. In fact, my clothes were feeling a bit looser than normal. I decide it was because I hadn't felt like eating as much. I also noticed the nausea subsiding and attributed it to finally making it over the hump.

Over the next week, I was feeling quite bothered by what happened on the river. I experienced some intense emotions and rage. My energy levels were increasing. I actually felt like going for a jog. It was odd. I hadn't felt much energy the entire pregnancy.

Back to the day I discovered her heart was no longer beating. I asked the doctor what was next. I was told that because of how far along I was, that there were many risks involved and that if she wasn't born soon, an infection could set in. My mind was spinning. I called Jacob. He was at the office adjusting patients. He immediately stopped everything and got in the car to come to us. I was an hour away as the midwife's office was several towns over. I was in no condition to be driving anywhere. The girls and I sat in the waiting room. Everything was closed as it was now after hours. The assistant stayed with us and gave us food and water. I was in shock. I called my sister and dad after trying my mom. I told them what happened. My mom phoned me and I told her. All three of them planned to immediately drive from Denver to Montrose and help in any way they can.

After what seemed like hours, Jacob arrived. We embraced. The sadness was overwhelming. Not knowing where we would go from there felt like too much. The unthinkable had happened. She was dead.

I called the midwife the following day, asking about what the options are. We decided that it was best to birth her as naturally as possible. The midwife would begin the process with a natural prostaglandin placed on the cervix to induce labor. I felt at peace with this route. I explained the environment we were used to having. She said she would make sure we had a safe and sacred space.

16

STILLBIRTH

An angel wrote down Finley's birth in the book of life and then whispered as she closed the book, "Too beautiful for Earth."

Two days after discovering I no longer had a live baby inside of me, Jacob, Grace and I were headed to the hospital to meet the midwife. It was 5:40 a.m. when we got up that morning. I showered, dressed and grabbed my snack bag, purse and journal. We headed to meet the midwife on the labor and delivery floor. I had never labored or delivered in a hospital before. I was nervous. This was definitely not what I'd envisioned for new baby's birth, surrounded by rooms that would usually be filled with moms at the end of their pregnancies, giving birth to full-size, live babies.

Here we were, entering into foreign territory to have a natural induction procedure so Finley Rose, who had died inside of me 2 weeks prior, could be born. To say this felt strange, is an understatement. I spent the next few moments looking around the room: the baby warmer in the corner, a large bed, a chair, a couch, shelving, a bathroom with tub, sinks and counter tops with cabinets full of supplies, a large baby heart monitor machine.

A nurse, Camille, entered the room with our midwife, Karen. Karen said they would make sure we have a safe and sacred space for today. Jacob basically laid it all out for them as far as his role and making sure no random people come into the room. He told them he had delivered all of our babies and this would be no different. Karen brought in the ultrasound machine. She turned it on and put it on my lower abdomen. Finley looked so squished compared with the other ultrasounds I had had over the past few weeks. Karen told us it was because amniotic fluid stopped being produced when the heart stops beating.

Finley Rose, you looked so tiny and cute and we could see your face and body. I knew it was time for you to come out. I had set a bedtime intention a couple nights prior, where I prayed for an answer regarding our next steps. I woke up the following morning knowing it was time and you wanted and needed to be born. Everything aligned for this to happen. It wasn't an easy decision I had to make. It was a self-honoring choice and your dad completely supported me in what needed to happen. Grace was really helpful. She played a major support role. She had been looking forward to Finley's birth all along. None of us knew it was going to be 22 weeks early.

Karen explained everything that would occur once the prostaglandins were placed behind my cervix. Jacob was the one who placed them there. The gel was cold. He put them in position. Karen and Camille left the room. Round 1. I felt tingling and tightening of my uterus. In preparation for birth, I'd put a few evening primrose capsules around my cervix to help with the softening. Today, my entire vaginal canal and the tissues surrounding the cervix are soft and fluffy. The cervical opening, however, is squeezed off and only 1 centimeter dilated. It feels puckered. I am thinking and visualizing opening. We made it the first 4 hours with not much of anything happening other than tightening of my uterus.

Round 2 started at 12:30 (round 1 was 8:30 a.m.). I kept questioning Camille: "How long will it take? What's the baby going to look like? How big will she be? Will there be something we can transport her home in?" I felt no pain or contractions and I was wondering if we would be there all day.

I write to her while sitting in the hospital bed:

> Finley Rose, I had no idea it was your death that caused me to feel so much better. I feel guilt about the fact that my feeling better was as a result of you dying. I love you. I love you . I love you. My love. You brought everyone so much joy. Your short life served great purpose in bringing our family closer and I am grateful to have been your mom. I will never forget the time I had with you. I love you, I love you, I love you. Thank you, Finley Rose for picking me. You completed your job, your task on this planet. We will miss you. I felt so much movement from you. And it was so early on that I began to feel you moving. I will remember you always.

Surely this would happen soon. Camille came in every so often to check on me. I told her nothing was happening yet. I kept feeling my belly and things were tightening. My uterus was in "clamp down" mode. Jacob and Grace went out to get lunch from Noodles. It was great to have a moment alone. I thought about what Finley would look like. What part of her would be born first? How big would she be? What would her face look like?

At 2:30 p.m. I did jumping jacks at Grace's suggestions. A minute later, my water broke. I was sitting up on the hospital bed and I jumped off and tons of bloody fluid splatted onto the ground. It was old blood, a burnt red color. We called in the nurse. She thought that everything would begin now.

We make it to Round 3. It's 4:30 p.m. More prostaglandins. This time I had Karen place them behind my cervix. Her fingers aren't as long as Jacob's and she had a harder time with it, but got it done fairly quickly. She told us it would be happening soon and that she would stay until 7 p.m. and then would have to leave.

I felt like nothing was getting anywhere. I could tell I wouldn't birth Finley by 7 p.m. All of my other experiences with birth had progressed more quickly than this. I did my best and stayed optimistic. I felt a drop inside of my lower abdomen. I was hopeful she'd come soon. Now my uterus was super tight and in my lower right abdomen, contracting away. We all started getting antsy. Grace had been rubbing my feet and legs and gave me a coloring book where you hunt for several objects and color them in. It was a welcomed distraction.

I was now bleeding and expelling clots like crazy. Karen came in just before she was to leave to check on me. Camille's shift was coming to a close at 8 p.m. Karen said it wouldn't be too much longer. She was sorry she wouldn't be there for the birth. She told us Dr. B would be helping us and that she knew about the details of our situation. Karen played a game with Grace and watched her making bracelets. She hugged us all goodbye.

Camille came in with the nurse that was taking over—Sierra. Sierra was young and very sweet. I asked her the same questions I'd already asked Camille and Karen and got the same answers. She told me, "When the birth does occur, it comes on quickly and you will most likely have the baby before anyone has a chance to do anything." She also said Finley would be the length of my hand or smaller and would have fully formed parts and pieces, very human-like.

I decided to get in the water. I started the bath and get the jets going. It was relaxing and I wondered why I hadn't done this earlier. I stayed in there almost an hour and got out to have some food.

At 8:30 Dr. B checked me. She was the first person that had ever done that other than myself or Jacob. She confirmed what I already knew, 1 centimeter. The uterus was moving downward though. Jacob put the capsules behind my cervix. At this point, I was thinking I would be there all night. I tried to sleep. I had painless, annoying contractions that wouldn't stop. They came on every few minutes and lasted for 1 minute.

Round 4 was doing something. I got up to go to the bathroom at 10 p.m. and felt something coming out. I reached down and felt the tiniest little arm and hand. I called Jacob in and he confirmed it was Finley's hand. We were both a bit taken aback and I wanted to see for myself. He took a picture of her hand. It looked just like your or my hand looks. Perfectly shaped fingers and the lines on her palm looked just like mine and she had crease lines on her fingers as well.

My cervix wasn't open enough for anything else to happen and I went back to bed. Jacob had hugged me in the hospital bed for an hour just after round 4 was administered. I really needed his support and could feel his love and Grace's love and caring.

At 11 p.m., I had to go the bathroom again. Her feet, legs and body easily slipped out. She looked gray and oxygen-depleted. I tried to push the rest of her out and she'd slide down a bit. I tried three or four more times and her head came out. She was caught by the "hat" resting on top of the toilet. We called the nurse. The cord was still attached. Jacob cut the cord. Sierra came in and grabbed Finley Rose and carefully laid her on a towel. I got off the toilet and got another pad set up so I could see her. Jacob was looking at her and it was clear to me what he was looking at. It looked as if she could be a boy. Dr. B came in and confirmed she was indeed a girl. Apparently it's normal at certain phases of development for the clitoris to look just like a penis.

Her hands were so tiny and perfect. Her elbows. Finley's shoulders looked strong. Her clavicles were the smallest I'd ever seen. Her ribcage was immaculate. Finley's belly had the tiniest bit of cut cord. Her little hips and knobby knees were so cute. Her ankles and feet had all the details of ankles and feet. Her toes were amazingly small and perfect. Her head was misshapen due to her skull bones not being developed enough to hold it all together. It made it difficult to make out what her face and head would look like if the structural integrity were there. I looked at her profile to get an idea. Her mouth was open and I could see her tongue. Her nostrils were the tiniest things on her and her nose was adorable. Her eyes were closed. Her ears were mashed close to her skull. Her skin and body had begun breaking down a couple of weeks ago, so not everything was as firm as usual. She was quite pliable.

Sierra spent a long time taking photos and molds for the memory box. We wrapped her in a blanket and took turns holding her and getting pictures. She measured 7 1/2 inches long. Her skin was slightly transparent. Grace put her treasured stuffed mouse in the blanket with Finley.

In the midst of all of this, I birthed the placenta shortly after Finley's birth. It came out in one big plop. Dr. B said it looked complete. I told her I wanted to go home. It was obvious they wanted us to stay awhile. However, she said I could go home after an hour if my bleeding was under control and it was. She was a very good doctor. She told me about her own experiences with miscarriage. Three times she went through miscarriages. She told me how she never gave herself time to heal, and that she could tell by my personality, I probably planned get right back into the office. She said to take at least two weeks. No matter what. Jacob had her repeat that to me. I told her I was feeling so amazing and could easily get back into the offices and my life. She went into more detail about her process and regrets when she miscarried. She was bleeding and performing surgeries. She said healing took forever because she was always on the go. She told me to tell patients with a message on our chalkboards, "We welcomed to the world, Finley Rose, born still, July 12th." I cannot tell you how impactful that was for me to hear about her personal experiences.

I knew I had to take the two weeks for healing. I made the self-honoring choice to do so, and I'm glad I did. It's incredible how many emotions and feelings and thoughts are running through your brain and body. Grace carried Finley out to the car after hugging Sierra and Dr. B goodbye. We drove home in the wee hours of the morning and our heads immediately hit the pillows upon entering our house.

I woke up sobbing. I remembered what had happened. In my sleep, I'd forgotten for a moment. It was as if nothing ever happened and I was still pregnant and she was alive. Jacob was right there, hugging me so tight. The grief coursed through me like a tidal wave. It was ready to take over and crash me onto the jagged rocks. Maybe this is what it would feel like if you were going to die. I was fully alive in that moment, feeling every sensation. I'd had so much happen that allowed me *to feel* those feelings. I let them pass through me and out of me. I did it again and again. My thoughts took me back to the accident on the river. Then to the ultrasound where I didn't hear her heartbeat. I couldn't see her moving. It all felt like too much. It felt like I was drowning. I prayed to God about Finley. Her life served a purpose. I was in acceptance of what had happened. I didn't like it, but I could accept it. She was there with me, an angel watching over us all. I felt her spirit. I knew we would make it through.

Two days later, we buried Finley Rose in the most beautiful place in the mountains. She has an outstanding view of the surrounding mountains and valleys. Jacob planted rose bushes and trees for her. Following the funeral, just as I had been journaling to her throughout my pregnancy, I wrote the following to her:

Finley Rose,

Your funeral was on Sunday, July 14th. You are in the most beautiful place and your daddy planted trees and rose bushes for you. We love you a lot. The girls and Daddy and I held you for the last time, inside the tiny home. You were wrapped in a beautiful white flower embroidered blanket. You were cold. I felt your feet. The toes. Grace's mouse was with you, keeping you company. Grace, Ada, Rae, Daddy and I cried and told you we loved you. We each had something for you. A letter from Grace and a letter from me. Bullets and coins from Daddy. A drawing from Ada and a drawing from Rae. Grace put a few more things in with you. Ada had a t-shirt for you that said, "A star is born." Daddy built you a beautiful pine box. It was smaller than a crate. We hugged and kissed you for the last time and Daddy nailed the pine box shut. We all prayed. We walked to the grave site. It's all really gorgeous. We all stood close together as Daddy began the service.

Our family and friends were there (25 of us total). Pastor Roberts gave a comforting message about where you were and how we'd see you in Heaven. Lots of Bible verses were read. Luke 12:7, Matthew 11:28-30, John 16:32, 1 John 5:4 and 2 Samuel 12.23. There's a lot of energy and emotion during the service. I held the girls close. Our family all crying and hugging. Lots of people said a few words. Grace read her letter to you, and I read my letter to you. At the end, we were all singing Amazing Grace as we dropped dirt over your pine box. Tons of white and pink roses were everywhere. We dropped the flowers over top of you. We love you more than you'll ever know. Afterwards we all headed to the cabin for food and drinks. Ada began sobbing during part of the funeral. I encouraged her and told her that it was okay to cry.

Here's the letter I wrote her:

Dear Finley Rose,

I am grateful for the time we had together. From the moment God blessed us with you, I loved you. I thank you for the gift you brought us. I miss you so much. Your kicks. Seeing you for the first time was incredible. We all enjoyed hearing your heart beating on the Doppler. Your tiny arms and legs wiggling around as if you were greeting us all. Your soul departed this earth far too soon for us. Your features are so perfectly formed and beautiful. I will always remember you and I look forward to playing with you in Heaven!

I love you with all my heart,
Your Mom

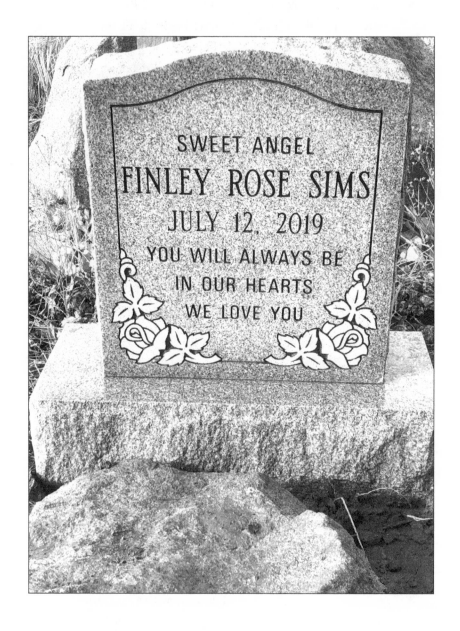

17

GOD SAYS YES

"Your heart knows the way.
Run in that direction."

-RUMI

I have learned a great deal from all of the experiences I've outlined in this book. I know there's more in store for our family. I do believe God has a plan here. I believe in the opportunities that will come as a result of everything I've just been through. In all truth, life feels really hard at times. I felt my mind going to some dark places following the loss of my unborn child—places of hopelessness where there is no light.

I recall one evening, I went out on our porch and looked up at the night sky. The stars looked alive that night. More vivid than usual. Her gravestone had just been delivered and was sitting on the front porch. I saw it and cried out to God. This was too painful. I looked up at the stars and I began thinking about what Finley would want. I knew she would want me to really live. She would want her parents to grow closer together. She would want me to infuse her beauty and light into everything. She wouldn't want me to isolate, fight, hurt or to be in fear. The fears that naturally arose in me regarding whether or not I choose to trust. For example: to trust in my body's ability to hold onto a pregnancy and birth a healthy child and to trust in God's plan for my life. Could I live in the present? Without infusing the past and/or negative future fantasies into it?

It feels impossible at times to implement the very things I know Finley came to teach me. She's taught me a lot about not taking anything for granted. She's taught me about what really matters. I've been on this journey of focusing on what really matters, and I find myself getting off track at times. The Thanksgiving following Finley's birth, as we talked about what we were grateful for, the girls all said they were thankful for our family and they listed every single one of us: "Dad, Mom, Grace, Ada and Rae Rae." Which reminded me of what my prayer with them is. Every night when I put them to bed, I thank God for each of us individually, listing it out just like they did. I add how I am grateful for all of our health.

The most precious thing in life is just that: life itself. Each of us brings a unique presence to the world. Every opportunity we are given is for our learning. Sometimes we are given similar challenges over and over again until we learn. Challenges bring growth.

I feel like throughout all of my experiences in life thus far, I've finally learned how to fill my cup on all levels—physically, mentally, emotionally and spiritually. This looks different for everyone. Following Finley's birth, I did weekly massages, adjustments, acupuncture, hot spring soaks, vapor caves, bible study, walks, therapy, date nights, "me time", journaling, lots of prayer and intention setting. I've continued do these things. This healing routine continues to make a big difference in my overall health.

Looking at the next season of life, I feel a strong calling for being involved in miscarriage support for other families experiencing what I've been through, to help others know that they aren't alone, know that recovery is possible, and to find the strength to live a life that honors that soul that was only here such a short time. I know serving in that capacity would help me just as much by finding purpose in tragedy. Following Finley's birth, I experienced support and love beyond anything I could have asked or imagined. I desire to give back. I want to serve others in that capacity. Whether it's in my everyday experiences where I can share my light with others, or in tragedy, where I can sit in the silence and be present with another human being where there are no words required. To be there with someone, just be—I see this as being part of my purpose in life. I did get inspired by a mentor of mine in the way of miscarriage support being part of my calling. It makes sense.

Winter arrived and I felt myself moving into the next season of life. Things had settled. The house felt peaceful. The routines of life felt lighthearted and trust was being restored. There was joy and zest for life, and a hope for the future. I experienced contentedness with where I was in life and with my family. I found myself saying things like, "I wouldn't have any regrets if I died today. My life has been filled with so much love. So many accomplishments and joyful experiences. The most fulfilling times revolve around my children."

I remember all of my pregnancies like they were yesterday—my baby bumps, the girls fluttering and moving around inside me, the excitement and anticipation of their births, and the beginning of labor. I remember not knowing how long it would take and how I felt I was going to be in labor for an eternity, and then having the urge to push. Right when I felt like throwing in the towel, I experienced a baby being born into the warm water, seeing them under the water, and then having them all immediately in my arms, watching them take their first breath. I can still see their faces, each one with a different expression. Grace had her eyes wide open, ready for anything. Ada's were closed and I remember her agitation with being outside of the womb. Rae was the largest of them all and she was so happy and content to be with all of us. Seeing into their soul through their eyes was magic. Each one so beautiful and innocent. I'll never forget what they all looked like as they breast fed all those years. The sweet sounds of contentedness, as they nursed. The immediate bonding that occurred between mother and child. Watching their dad be softened by his daughters. It's incredible to see the man you love be absolutely transformed by a tiny baby.

My life feels completely transformed in ways I cannot put into words. Nor could I have predicted any of it. I remember when we were first dating and we talked about how big of a family we each wanted. He said he wanted three kids and I said I wanted to have four kids. Then, after Grace was born and I wasn't getting much sleep, I told my husband I think one is enough... Clearly God had other plans. The feeling just swept over me and I realized when Grace was 18 months old that I most definitely was ready for another. Our sweet Ada was born and I knew I wasn't finished. Then Rae came along. She infused a joy into our family like nothing else we'd experienced up to that point. Then, we had Finley coming and I really couldn't believe that my initial prediction was happening.

I had many thoughts about having another baby. Do I want to do that again? My initial thoughts were, "why would I ever put myself in that position ever again!". It felt impossible to even think about getting pregnant. I felt the need for more healing. I wondered if it was even possible. How can I trust that everything won't crumble around me in the event I conceive and have something tragic take place, yet again?

I'm much stronger now than I've ever been. In some ways, I feel invincible. I think about my girls and what would happen if they experienced another huge let down. I don't want them to be let down ever again. I also want them to experience the joys of a new baby. The door is definitely not closed on the idea. Regardless of all of the pain and trauma I've recently experienced, I can see myself experiencing conception, pregnancy, birth and holding a new baby in my arms.

I've forgiven myself for judgements I have surrounding Finley, any feelings of guilt or regret that I could have done anything differently. I feel like my physical being is healed. I gave myself permission to feel joy again, permission to put my heart on the line again, permission to think about the opportunities that have come as a result of that experience, permission to make more memories. I feel the freedom and lightness in my day to day. I have renewed trust and faith in God's plan here.

And wouldn't you know it, despite the fact that we aren't trying, another surprise in store! I'm pregnant!

ACKNOWLEDGEMENTS

Thank you to my husband, my rock throughout all of my pregnancies and births. Thank you for loving me.

Thank you to my mom for the example you set for natural birth back when you had me and it wasn't the popular thing to do.

Thank you to Drs. Ron and Mary Hulnick, as well as the entire USM community, for the love and support in completing this book.

ABOUT
THE AUTHOR

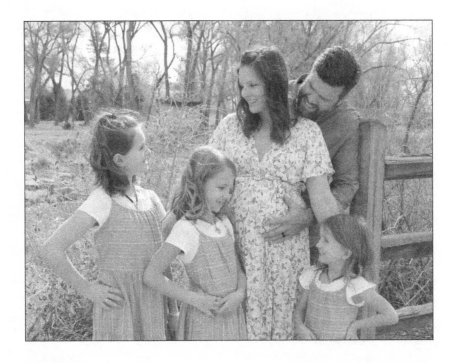

Dr. Laura Sims has been helping people reach optimal health since 2006. Along with her husband, they founded 2 of the largest chiropractic practices on the western slope of Colorado.

She believes the body is capable of healing itself when free from nerve interference. In 2019, she completed a 2-year Master's class in Soul-Centered Living from the University of Santa Monica. It is her heartfelt mission for everyone to step more fully into their courageousness and trust their inner knowing!

Her personal affirmations:

I am fully accepting all parts of myself, generously sharing my beauty and love with myself and others.

I am peacefully living in full trust of myself and others, authentically expressing my joyful creativity.

Ideal Scene for Radiant Health Throughout Pregnancy:

- *I am fully accepting my appearance*
- *I am radiating light and love*
- *I am fully embracing myself*
- *I am gracious with myself*
- *I am in integrity and vulnerable*
- *I am sleeping soundly, all night long*
- *I am feeling bountiful every*
- *I am taking care of all of my needs*
- *I am enjoying the process and sharing updates with my family daily*
- *I am mentally, emotionally, physically and spiritually preparing for an amazing, smooth, speedy birth*
- *I ask for what I need*
- *I am delegating tasks and lightening my load*

Living Vision:

I wake up feeling fully rested and full of light, excited for the day. I'm jumping out of bed and hugging Jacob and the girls. I'm greeting the day with vibrancy and I'm enjoying my morning tea and juice. Yum! This is after my yoga practice or walking/running and my body feels so alive. Every cell is vibrating on a high frequency and I'm feeling ecstatic about my life. I am in complete gratitude as I interact with the girls and Jacob. I feel so happy with myself and my family. Thank you God for this incredible life! I am interacting with everyone around me and feeling on top of the world. All of my patients are experiencing healing coming through me (conduit of God's healing). I am re energized after eating nutritious food that feels amazing. The afternoon is full of experiences I take on with grace and ease. When I get back home, I'm having loving interactions with the girls and we eat a delicious home-cooked dinner together. I greet the night and jump into bed, reading books that make me feel empowered and invigorated. Pray. Night Night...